Defining Multiple Chemical Sensitivity

ALSO BY BONNYE L. MATTHEWS:

*Chemical Sensitivity: A Guide to Coping
with Hypersensitivity Syndrome, Sick Building
Syndrome and Other Environmental Illnesses*
(McFarland, 1992)

Defining Multiple Chemical Sensitivity

Edited by

Bonnye L. Matthews

McFarland & Company, Inc., Publishers

Jefferson, North Carolina, and London

British Library Cataloguing-in-Publication data are available

Library of Congress Cataloguing-in-Publication Data

Defining multiple chemical sensitivity / edited by Bonnye L.
    Matthews.
        p.   cm.
    Includes bibliographical references and index.
    ISBN 0-7864-0413-2 (library binding : 50# alkaline paper)
    1. Multiple chemical sensitivity.   I. Matthews, Bonnye L.,
    1943–   .
    [DNLM: 1. Multiple Chemical Sensitivity.   2. Environmental
    Exposure — adverse effects.   3. Occupational Exposure — adverse
    effects.   4. Occupational Diseases — chemically induced.   WA 30.5
    D313   1998]
    RB152.6.D44   1998
    615.9'02 — dc21
    DNLM/DLC
    for Library of Congress   98-3762
                                                                          CIP

Manufactured in the United States of America

McFarland & Company, Inc., Publishers
  Box 611, Jefferson, North Carolina 28640

To Gordon P. Baker, M.D.

CONTENTS

Contents

PREFACE

When I wrote *Chemical Sensitivity* (McFarland, 1992), I had in mind a book that would inform. It is well that I had no other goal in mind. Had I even suspected the response that came, I would have been terrified to begin. Many letters and cards and phone calls from chemical sensitives assured me that the book had had great meaning for them. Several contacted me with the message that the book had destroyed their plan for suicide. I was moved. Such an objective for the book was so far from my thoughts that I hardly knew how to respond.

A few doctors found amusement over my lengthy bibliography. I responded with fact: my subject was science and medicine. Interestingly, some of the doctors who work against recognition of chemical sensitivity as a real (as opposed to psychogenic) illness or disease had some very positive comments regarding the book. Reviewers' assessments of the book tended to be based on the degree to which chemical sensitivity related to them. Glowing reports came from those who are environmentally aware. One repeated criticism was that I was writing a book on a subject for which I was not credentialed, though this complaint was accompanied by little or no evidence of an effort to determine whether the information was nevertheless accurate and appropriate.

Why another book? A few reasons: (1) New medical information has come to light that explains certain cases of chemical sensitivity as already recognized diseases; this information will not hit the medical journals for a time (I write in February 1998) but people need to be informed about it. (2) I have found professionals to deal with the medical information and legal information which is not easily accessible to many. And (3) I am convinced that most of the public has no idea what happens to a person who develops chemical sensitivity, so I aim to make that clear.

The book is divided into four sections, each looking at chemical sensitivity from a different angle. Section I is recent medical information.

Section II gives an idea of the current legal picture. Section III takes a look at some of the literature often cited as "proof" that MCS is a manifestation of psychiatric disorder. Section IV is an overview of my own experience with chemical sensitivity.

As it was with the first book, my purpose is to inform. This time the depth is greater. It is possible that a reader unacquainted with those who have been chemically injured may find some of this information unbelievable. The expression "truth is stranger than fiction" is no news to the chemically injured or those who treat or advocate for them. The environment in which all this activity takes place is hidden from mainstream life.

I have personally been acquainted with two chemically injured individuals who committed suicide. Over 100 other MCS-related suicides are known. What surprises me is not that they did but rather that more have not. The stress placed on these sick people is severe. What is amazing to me still is the number of them who work so desperately to prevent others from a fate such as theirs.

I was poisoned in 1987 and discovered it in 1988 following an explosive reaction. I was in my forties. Despite my age I was very naive. Since then I've picked up the rocks and looked underneath. By rocks I mean the reasons why there is such strong resistance to formally recognizing the disorder. Why do MCS sufferers encounter such stressful opposition? I have found ugly things under those rocks, really ugly things. I have gone through shock at seeing them. I have experienced anger, even rage. I have asked the usual questions, "How could they?" "How dare they?"

They can as long as the general public has no idea what occurs. Like growing numbers of others, I know what happens to the chemically injured. As long as I am able, I, like they, will continue to inform. The truth is that with information this disease does not have to occur. Not one more individual need be transformed by what for many is total and permanent disability.

I

MEDICAL INFORMATION

The first three chapters of this section are the work of professionals who have first-hand knowledge of chemical injury. Each is or has been involved in the treatment of numbers of chemically injured patients. These professionals do not necessarily know each other or share the same perspectives. Yet they do have at least one thing in common: Each recognizes that chemical injury causes real and sometimes lethal damage.

Chapter 4 examines what may be the single most significant finding in recent years, namely that many chemical sensitivities have a recognized disease known as porphyria. This disease involves the metabolism of heme, a component of hemoglobin. (Hemoglobin aids in the attachment of oxygen to blood cells.) Though medical science has long been acquainted with porphyria (also known as porphyrinopathy or porphyrin abnormality), it was previously thought to be a rare, inherited condition. The discovery that ordinary chemical exposure can induce porphyria has profound implications, not only for treatment, but for the way MCS is perceived by the medical community.

1. CHEMICAL SENSITIVITY: A PSYCHOLOGICAL PERSPECTIVE

Eileen R. McCarty

It is not only computer knowledge and technology that has exploded in recent years. Research in general has moved to new heights, in new directions, and across scientific and environmental disciplines. As always, certain developments are born of necessity to explain identified phenomena. The growing quantity of information about chemical sensitivity is no exception.

In 1983, Bernard Weiss[1] stated that the adverse impact of environmental chemicals should be gauged by how people feel and function, not solely by death or overt damage. This timely challenge went largely unheeded. Industries continued to use powerful chemicals, choosing to focus on how well the substances worked in the manufacture of products or the control of agricultural pests. Focus on human functional deficits and impairments, or on the identification of new illnesses that might be related to exposure to the chemicals, continued to be secondary.

Meanwhile, chemically exposed individuals experienced difficulty with memory and concentration, or perhaps felt fatigued. Often these subtle symptoms were shrugged off as stress related. When symptoms intensified and were complicated by respiratory and gastrointestinal illnesses, victims began to seek medical help. By now, many individuals were experiencing collections of symptoms that crossed systems, as well as recognized illnesses defined by the presence of certain symptom clusters.

Because victims of chemical exposure often felt better during weekends or short vacations (when most of them were removed from the presence of offending chemicals), it took time to establish that chemical air pollution causes permanent impairments over time, even when exposure is indirect, lower level or intermittent. Most exposed individuals simply sought treatment for predominant symptoms and returned to work. Later in the progression of their illness, however, many victims became aware that not only was the workplace toxic, but the route to work, with its vehicle exhaust, was likewise a threat. Even the typical household, full of cleaning agents, perfumes, deodorants and hair sprays, was a dangerous environment. Victims learned to direct their efforts toward cleaning their personal environments and detoxifying their bodies. Some attained a measure of relief. Some found their "symptoms" reclassified as permanent impairments.

Psychological evaluation of exposed individuals revealed variation in cognitive and emotional symptoms as well as reported physical symptoms. Intensity of symptoms varied. Function was more impaired immediately after departure from the toxic environment than it was several months later.

Several factors suggested that susceptibility to damage from chemical exposure may vary. Some individuals were exposed for longer periods than others. Some chemicals appeared to be more potent than others. Not all individuals had the same level of intellectual ability or emotional stability prior to illness. There was no homogeneity in personality style. From a clinical perspective, the psychologist found a shifting of outcomes for a single individual and across individuals.

To complicate diagnostic identification, some cognitive impairments due to industrial toxins proved difficult to measure by standard psychological instruments. Murial Lezak[2] established that executive functions — abilities to formulate goals, to plan, and to carry out plans effectively — were impaired. Difficulties in these areas were detected through interview data — often in the recital of "things I used to do but can no longer do" — or through significant errors in daily activity. Lezak[3] identified some neuropsychological tests as helpful in detecting impairment in groups of brain-impaired individuals.

The picture seemed ever more complex, making it difficult to acquire complete data and to form the hypotheses needed to examine the damaging process of exposure to chemicals. Litigation, and perhaps the reluctance of professionals to accept the existence of such an elusive phenomenon, muddied the path of progress.

Although collating data from more specific and well-defined study samples has helped to identify symptoms directly related to chemical sensitivity, it is difficult to isolate symptoms when individuals present with a myriad of problem areas crossing body systems. With time, research has focused on understanding how chemicals permeate and affect the central nervous system. Because of ethical considerations and the potential for damage, data are often gleaned from animal studies and from study of individuals affected by environmental and industrial accidents. Metabolic imaging studies by Callender et al.[4] have shown abnormal SPECT brain scans in individuals with a clinical diagnosis of toxic encephalopathy after exposure to neurotoxins. Synthesizing information about chemical sensitivity from various disciplines, Bell, Miller and Schwartz[5] have developed an olfactory-limbic model of chemical sensitivity which offers an explanation for reaction to low levels of inhaled and ingested chemicals that result in persistent cognitive, emotional, and somatic symptoms.

Recently, people with known toxic encephalopathy have tested positive for acute intermittent porphyria. Once considered a rare hereditary disease,[6] this illness is now occurring in persons with no family history. Acute intermittent porphyria is a complex illness related to deficient enzyme activity in the biosynthetic pathway of heme. Exposure to a variety of drugs and chemicals is known to induce porphyria, which can cause both neurological symptoms (such as peripheral neuropathy and sensory disorder) and central nervous system symptoms (such as anxiety, depression, and confusion). The only treatment is avoidance of precipitant chemicals and drugs and adherence to a vegetarian diet high in carbohydrates.

Recent evidence suggests that DHEA (dehydroepiandrosterone), a steriod hormone produced in the adrenal gland, needs replacing when it falls too low in the body. Exposure to certain chemicals seems to hasten the decline of DHEA production. Replacement of DHEA at the proper dosage appears to improve energy and clarify thought processes. An individual will still likely react to chemical exposure, but his or her overall quality of life may be enhanced.

Sometimes the search for answers leads only to further questions; passing through one door, we discover more doors waiting to be opened. In the matter of chemical sensitivity, we have yet to find a universal explanation. What is true for one patient may not apply to another — and what is true for the non-sensitive individual may not apply to the chemically sensitive. An exposed patient may look or sound like someone suffering from emotional or mental illness, but, the fit may be only superficial. It would behoove clinicians not to move too quickly to diagnosis. The patient is entitled to that respect.

Because the chemically sensitive patient is often referred to a variety of specialists, he or she needs a primary physician to function as an orchestra leader. Keeping the data straight, as well as reviewing and balancing the treatment options, is important. The exposed individual probably has neither the broad background nor (at least at time of exposure) the emotional stability to keep the facts straight.

Perhaps a very significant factor in the cognitive and emotional aspects of chemical sensitivity is that the symptom list is endless. Some symptoms are specific to chemical sensitivity. Others are prompted by the individual's response to the injury, which is a function of his or her personality structure as shaped by experience. Still others are the result of adaptation to an altered self. The clinician has the opportunity and challenge to guide in the process of understanding, accepting and adapting. The clinician also has the opportunity to educate the community about chemical sensitivity and to increase awareness about self-protection from exposure.

In this vein, a colleague reported to me that a cosmetic salesperson related her poorly adhering nail polish to the lessening or removal of formaldehyde in the formula. Progress is evident on many fronts.

References

1. B. Weiss, "Behavioral Toxicology and Environmental Health Science: Opportunity and Challenge for Psychology," *American Psychologist* **38** (1983): 1174–1187.

2. M. Lezak, "Neuropsychologist Assessment in Behavioral Toxicology: Developing Techniques and Interpretive Issues," undated paper, Veterans Administration Medical Center and Oregon Health Sciences University.

3. M. Lezak, *Neurological Assessment*, 2nd edition (New York: Oxford University Press, 1983).

4. T. Callender, L. Morrow, K. Subramanian, D. Duhon, and M. Ristovv, "Three-dimensional Brain Metabolic Imaging in Patients with Toxic Encephalopathy," *Environmental Research* **60** (1993): 295–319.

5. I. Bell, C. Miller, and G. Schwartz, "An Olfactory-Limbic Model of Multiple Chemical Sensitivity Syndrome: Possible Relationships to Kindling and Affective Spectrum Disorders," *Biological Psychiatry* **32** (1992): 218–242.

6. W. Massey, "Neuropsychiatric Manifestations of Porphyria," *Journal of Clinical Psychiatry* **41** (1980): 208–213.

2. MCS: TRIAL BY SCIENCE

Donald L. Dudley, M.D.

The olfactory system has received only marginal attention in the search for possible initiators of Multiple Chemical Sensitivity (MCS). This is in keeping with the medical community's general lack of interest in the olfactory system, which has never represented a popular or fashionable area of research for most investigators. This attitude has been present for at least a century[1] and has been perpetuated by prestigious textbooks.[2] Thus research in the olfactory system has lagged behind our explorations of the auditory and visual systems (which are actually less complex). As a result, the research community has failed to establish the groundwork needed for the diagnosis and treatment of MCS and other diseases.

Mother Nature appears to hold the olfactory system in greater esteem, providing backup connections or systems in the brain to protect it. Parts of the olfactory system can be altered or even deleted without significant harm.[3] Some writers have pointed to this fact as proof that the system has little value, but in fact the opposite is true; damage can be accommodated because the system is so well supported and protected, just as the Circle of Willis protects the arterial blood supply to the brain.

Olfactory receptors occupy only two square centimeters and consist of 6 million receptor cells in the dorsal aspect of the nasal cavity, the septum and part of the superior turbinates. These receptor cells are true neurons, but unlike other neurons they are not static. They undergo continual turnover throughout life. The lifespan of each cell appears to be between 30 and 210 days, with complete turnover of cells every six weeks. The olfactory receptors have four primary functions: (1) to detect odors from chemical stimuli; (2) to transduce information regarding the identity of the chemical as well as its concentration and the time of stimulation; (3) to couple this information to the electrical properties of the neuron; (4) to transmit this information to the brain.

Most studies of chemical toxicity have focused on the immune system. This focus has produced much contradictory and hard-to-interpret information.[4,5] Thus, despite the vigor of arguments both for and against the existence of MCS, there has been no scientific basis for either position.

It was this author's feeling that focusing on the olfactory system — whose work is electrochemical and not directly related to immunology — might prove more productive. The present study therefore quantifies the cognitive and somatosensory evoked potentials, which appropriately represent the electrochemical nature of the system being studied.

MATERIAL AND METHODS

Twenty patients with severe chemical sensitivity, who fulfilled the criteria for MCS as published by Cullen,[8] were studied. They were the first 20 patients who fulfilled the criteria and were not otherwise selected. All were former full-time employees who had to stop work because of chemical sensitivity. Half were self-referred and half were referred by an attorney or physician. All had been treated unsuccessfully by five or more physicians and were feeling desperate. There were five males and fifteen females between the ages of 33 and 60, with a mean age of 44 and a median age of 43. These people were unable to perform the activities of daily living when exposed to chemicals. Their problems with chemical odors were of a magnitude that this author had not previously seen.

Among the measurements recorded were psychophysical ratings relative to patients' ability to function when away from offending chemicals for at least one week and then following exposure for a minimum of 30 minutes. (For methodology of this type of measurement see Stevens.[9]) A rating of zero represented normal intellectual, emotional and physical functions, and a rating of 10 represented the most impairment in the same functions the patient had ever experienced. Intermediate ratings were linear; a rating of 5 represented 50 percent of the impairment and 2 represented 20 percent. Both author and patients considered a rating of 0 to 4 compatible with work. All patients were required to supply informed consent, although they considered exposure in the laboratory to be no different from exposure they regularly experienced.

The author considered the study an "experiment of nature" since all chemical exposure was done with chemicals the patients felt they were sensitive to and brought to the laboratory themselves. There were 18 different sensitivities reported:

> 11 patients were sensitive to perfume
> 8 were sensitive to felt tip pens
> 6 were sensitive to carpet adhesive
> 6 were sensitive to formaldehyde
> 5 were sensitive to polyurethane preservative
> 4 were sensitive to silicone sealant
> 3 were sensitive to window cleaner
> 3 were sensitive to paint
> 2 were sensitive to gasoline
> 2 were sensitive to copy machine toner
> 2 were sensitive to paint primer
> 2 were sensitive to wood stain
> 2 were sensitive to a concrete bonding agent
> 2 were sensitive to methyl ethyl ketone
> 1 was sensitive to acetone
> 1 was sensitive to floor stripper
> 1 was sensitive to nail polish
> and 1 was sensitive to diesel fuel

The exposures were standardized as much as possible by placing the chemicals on a small glass or stainless steel tray placed three feet from the patient. All told, 62 chemicals were used in exposure. Each patient had an average of exposure to more than three chemicals. The purpose was not to standardize the chemicals, but to find out if these people were having a reaction that could be objectively measured. The amount of chemical varied from three to four milliliters to simply opening a felt tip pen and waving it near the patient; a "correct" amount was determined by whether the patient could smell it. In some cases the author had a hard time knowing if the patient was exposed since he could not smell the chemical himself and had to depend on the patient's reports. Standardization was felt to be present in that each patient was exposed to the chemicals he or she felt were causing problems. It was the author's opinion that the carriers in most of the products and some of the individual chemicals fit the description in the literature of excitatory amino acid agonists.[10]

Neurometric testing was done prior to and following 30 minutes of exposure to the chemical. Exposure was maintained as long as testing continued. Prior to testing and during the control (prior to the 30-minute exposure) the laboratory air was exchanged every four minutes to be certain there were no extraneous smells in the laboratory. The air was drawn from the adjoining hallway, which was an area where no patient complained of undesirable chemicals. A Cadwell-32 was used to measure the evoked potentials.[11]

Visual evoked potentials are electrophysiologic responses of the retina and optical pathways to electromagnetic waves in the visual range. Auditory evoked potentials are responses of the auditory nerve to acoustic stimulation in the receptor range. In the present study, the visual stimulus was a reversing checkerboard screen operating at two cycles per second. The auditory stimulus was a series of clicking sounds played several times per second through headphones.

Visual and auditory evoked or "event-related" potentials (ERPs) are easily measured by means of noninvasive electrical recordings from the scalp. Scalp-recorded ERPs are analyzed as a series of positive and negative voltages that occur at predictable times. Longer-latency components are referred to as the cognitive evoked potential (cognitive EP) or endogenous ERPs.

The P300 (P3 or cognitive EP) is a well-known endogenous ERP. *It is known not to be influenced by emotional factors.* Others in this category include earlier waves known as N1, P2 and N2.[12,13] In the present study the ERPs, which were measured in the right and left ear and right and left eye independently, were mapped on a spectrum of 21 standard electroencephalographic electrodes. For purposes of clarity, in this paper, a single standard electrode (CZ or number 11) was used to present the data. Electrode 11 is one of the electrodes traditionally used for presentation of evoked potential information and is significantly correlated with electrodes FZ and PZ, which are the other electrodes used for quantification of P300. All measurements were identical to standard measurements made in other laboratories.

The P300 is the most widely studied ERP. It is the largest ERP component and is consistently positive in polarity with a 300- to 400-millisecond latency after the occurrence of an infrequent stimulus (rare or oddball stimulus) to which the patient is attending. The P300 has been correlated with the speed at which sequential decisions can be made, suggesting that it is generated by neural systems involved in the decision-making process. The P300 latency voltage (amplitude) is increased as the rare stimulus becomes rarer. The latency is increased with increasing task difficulty or complexity of stimulus evaluation.[12,13] These observations are relative. For example a patient with Alzheimer's disease to whom a simple task is complex will have a longer latency.[14]

The n (number) for the auditory ERPs in this study is 20. The n (number) for the visual ERPs is 18 rather than 20 because the checkerboard screen was not functioning while two patients were being chemically exposed.

The study also measured responses to electrical stimulation in the median nerve (Upper SSEP or USSEP) and the posterior tibial nerve (Lower SSEP or LSSEP). The stimulus was a square-wave electrical pulse of 100 microsecond duration, 5–30 volts and 5–30 milliamps (depending on the adequacy of the response).

The ERPs for the USSEP are called the N19 and P22. The N19 is widely recognized as the signal at the thalamus and the P22 at the primary somatosensory cortex. The ERPs for the LSSEP are called the P37 and N45. The P37 is recognized as the signal at the primary sensory cortex and the N45 to represent the signal at higher cortical centers. They were measured at CZ or PZ and as universally standardized.

The statistical approach involved paired samples and linear regression and correlation, using the computer programs produced by Glantz.[15] The selection of the statistical methods was in accordance with the selection methods in his computer program.

RESULTS

Table I
Right Auditory (n = 20) and Visual (n = 18) P300R Latency Before and During Chemical Stimulation

Right P300R Before		320.15 ms
Auditory	$T = 5.83$	$p = <0.0001$
Right P300R During		437.65 ms
Right P300R Before		430.39 ms
Visual	$T = 3.36$	$p = <0.004$
Right P300R During		497.33 ms

[13]

As illustrated in Table I, the latency of the right auditory P300 at electrode 11 (CZ) was 320 milliseconds (ms) prior to chemical exposure. During chemical exposure, latency at the same position was 438 ms. This change is significant, p = <0.0001. The mean latency of the right visual P300 at electrode 11 was 430 ms prior to exposure. The mean latency during chemical exposure was 497 ms. This is significant, p = <0.004.

Table II
Right Auditory (n = 20) and Visual (n = 18) P300R Amplitude
Before and During Chemical Stimulation

Right P300R Before	13.39 mv	
Auditory	T = 5.04	p = <0.0001
Right P300R During	7.79 mv	
Right P300R Before	9.51 mv	
Visual	T = 0.50	p = <0.62
Right P300R During	9.06 mv	

As illustrated in Table II, the amplitude of the right auditory P300 was 13.4 microvolts (mv) prior to chemical exposure. During chemical exposure the amplitude was 7.8 mv. This reduction in amplitude is significant, p = <0.0001. The amplitude of the right visual P300 was 9.5 mv prior to chemical exposure. During chemical exposure, amplitude was 9.1 mv. This is not significant, p = <0.62.

Table III
Right Upper SSEP Latency
Before and During Olfactory Stimulation (n = 18)

N19 Before Stimulation	19.5 ms	
Right Latency	T = 5.72	p = <0.0001
N19 During Stimulation	22.2 ms	
P22 Before Stimulation	23.1 ms	
Right Latency	T = 3.22	p = <0.005
P22 During Stimulation	26.8 ms	

Table III shows the right USSEP latency before and during chemical exposure. The N19 was 19.5 before exposure and 22.2 during exposure. This increase in latency was significant, p = <0.0001. The right P22 was 23.1 ms prior to exposure and 26.8 ms during exposure. This increase was significant at p = <0.005.

Table IV
Right Upper SSEP Amplitude Before and
During Olfactory Stimulation (n = 18)

N19 Before Stimulation		2.5 mv
Right Amplitude	T = 2.22	p = <0.04
N19 During Stimulation		1.2 mv
P22 Before Stimulation		3.8 mv
Right Amplitude	T = 1.25	p = <0.23
P22 During Stimulation		2.1 mv

Table IV shows the right USSEP amplitude before and during chemical exposure. The right N19 was 2.5 mv before exposure and 1.2 during exposure. This was significant at p = <0.04. The right P22 was 3.8 mv before chemical exposure and 2.1 mv during exposure. This was not significant, p = <0.23.

Table V
Right Lower SSEP Latency Before and
During Olfactory Stimulation (n = 18)

P37 Before Stimulation		39.0 ms
Right Latency	T = 2.65	p = <0.02
P37 During Stimulation		43.7 ms
N45 Before Stimulation		46.4 ms
Right Latency	T = 3.36	p = <0.004
N45 During Stimulation		50.7 ms

Table V shows the latency of the right LSSEP before and during chemical exposure. The right P37 latency was 39.0 ms before exposure and 43.7 ms during exposure. This was significant, p = <0.02. The right N45 latency was 46.4 ms prior to chemical exposure and 50.7 ms during exposure. This was significant, p = <0.004.

Table VI
Right Lower SSEP Amplitude Before and
During Olfactory Stimulation (n = 18)

P37 Before Stimulation		3.0 mv
Right Amplitude	T = 0.68	p = <0.51
P37 During Stimulation		2.5 mv

[15]

Table VI (cont.)

N45 Before Stimulation		3.7 mv
Right Amplitude	T = 1.16	p = <0.26
N45 During Stimulation		2.9 mv

Table VI shows the amplitude of the LSSEP prior to and during chemical exposure. The right P37 was 3.0 mv prior to exposure and 2.5 mv during exposure. This was not significant, p = <0.51. The right N45 was 3.7 mv before exposure and 2.9 mv during exposure. This was not significant, p = <0.26.

Table VII
Left Auditory (n = 20) and Visual (n = 18) P300R Latency
Before and During Chemical Stimulation

Left P300R Before		343.30 ms
Auditory	T = 4.94	p = <0.0001
Left P300R During		470.85 ms
Left P300R Before		413.83 ms
Visual	T = 3.37	p = <0.004
Left P300R During		509.78 ms

As illustrated in Table VII, the latency of the left auditory P300 was 343 ms prior to chemical exposure and 471 ms during exposure. This was significant, p = <0.0001. The mean latency of the left visual P300 was 414 ms prior to exposure and 510 ms during exposure. This was significant, p = <0.004.

Table VIII
Left Auditory (n = 20) and Visual (n = 18) P300R Amplitude
Before and During Chemical Exposure

Left P300R Before		11.82 mv
Auditory	T = 4.087	p = <0.0001
Left P300R During		2.20 mv
Left P300R Before		9.00 mv
Visual	T = 0.65	p = <0.53
Left P300R During		8.43 mv

Table VIII shows the amplitude of the left auditory P300 to be 11.8 mv prior to exposure and 2.2 mv during exposure. This was significant, p = <0.0001. The mean amplitude of the left visual P300 was 9.0 mv prior to exposure and 8.4 mv during exposure. This was not significant, p = <0.53.

Table IX
Left Upper SSEP Latency Before and During
Olfactory Stimulation (n = 18)

N19 Before Stimulation		18.7 ms
Left Latency	T = 4.32 p = <0.0001	
N19 During Stimulation		22.2 ms
P22 Before Stimulation		22.7 ms
Left Latency	T = 3.58 p = <0.003	
P22 During Stimulation		29.3 ms

Table IX shows the left USSEP latency before and during chemical exposure. The N19 latency was 18.7 ms before and 22.2 ms during exposure. This increase in latency was significant, p = <0.0001. The P22 was 22.7 ms prior to stimulation and 29.3 ms during stimulation. This augmentation of latency was significant, p = <0.003.

Table X
Left Upper SSEP Amplitude Before and During
Olfactory Stimulation (n = 18)

N19 Before Stimulation		2.5 mv
Left Amplitude	T = 2.22 p = <0.04	
N19 During Stimulation		1.2 mv
P22 Before Stimulation		3.8 mv
Left Amplitude	T = 1.25 p = <0.23	
P22 During Stimulation		2.1 mv

Table X shows the left USSEP amplitude before and during chemical exposure. The N19 amplitude was 2.5 mv prior to exposure and 1.2 mv during exposure. This was significant, p = <.04. The P22 amplitude was 3.8 mv before exposure and 2.1 mv during exposure. This was not significant, p = <0.23.

Table XI
Left Lower SSEP Latency Before and During Olfactory Stimulation (n = 18)

P37 Before Stimulation		38.7 ms
Left Latency	T = 4.61 p = <0.002	
P37 During Stimulation		47.2 ms
N45 Before Stimulation		47.4 ms
Left Latency	T = 3.71 p = <0.002	
N45 During Stimulation		55.0 ms

Table XI shows the LSSEP latency before and during chemical exposure. The P37 before and during exposure was 38.7 and 47.2 ms respectively. This was significant at $p = <0.0001$. The N45 latency before and during exposure was 47.4 and 55.0 ms respectively. This was significant, $p = <0.002$.

Table XII
Left Lower SSEP Amplitude Before and During Olfactory Stimulation (n = 19)

P37 Before Stimulation		4.8 mv
Left Amplitude	T = 1.77 p = <0.26	
P37 During Stimulation		2.0 mv
N45 Before Stimulation		3.9 mv
Left Amplitude	T = 2.21 p = <0.04	
N45 During Stimulation		2.1 mv

Table XII shows the LSSEP amplitude before and during chemical exposure. The P37 before and during exposure was 4.8 mv and 2.0 mv respectively. This was not significant, $p = <0.26$. The N45 before and during exposure was 3.9 mv and 2.1 mv respectively. This was significant, $p = <.04$.

Table XIII
Correlation of Right and Left Auditory and Visual P300R Latency Prior to and During Chemical Exposure

Auditory (n = 20) prior to	R = 0.08	T = 0.33	p = <0.75
Auditory (n = 20) during	R = 0.72	T = 4.37	p = <0.0001
Visual (n = 18) prior to	R = 0.42	T = 1.83	p = <0.09
Visual (n = 18) during	R = 0.70	T = 3.95	p = <0.001

The data were also analyzed for correlations between pre-exposure and post-exposure readings. As illustrated in Table XIII, the auditory P300 latencies in the right and left ears do not correlate prior to exposure, r = 0.08 and p = <0.75. However, during exposure there is a high correlation, r = 0.72 and p = <0.0001. The visual P300 latencies in the right and left eyes also do not correlate prior to exposure, r = 0.42 and p = <0.09. However, during exposure the correlation is high, r = 0.70 and p = <0.001.

Table XIV
Correlation of Right and Left Auditory and Visual P300R Amplitude Prior to and During Chemical Exposure

Auditory (n = 20) prior to	R = 0.82	T = 5.69	p = <0.0001
Auditory (n = 20) during	R = 0.66	T = 3.77	p = <0.001
Visual (n = 18) prior to	R = 0.93	T = 10.36	p = <0.0001
Visual (n = 18) during	R = 0.75	T = 4.47	p = <0.001

As illustrated in Table XIV, the correlation of amplitude goes in the opposite direction; the p value increases and the r value falls. The correlation of right and left auditory amplitudes before exposure is 0.82 (p = <0.0001), during exposure r = 0.66 and p = <0.001. The correlation of the right and left visual P300 amplitudes before exposure is 0.93 (p = <0.0001). During exposure the correlation is 0.75 (p = <0.001).

Table XV
Correlation of Right and Left Upper SSEP Latency Prior to and During Chemical Exposure

N19 Latency prior to	R = 0.05	T = 0.20	p = <0.85
N19 Latency during	R = 0.42	T = 1.87	p = <0.08
P22 Latency prior to	R = 0.18	T = 0.70	p = <0.50
P22 Latency during	R = 0.67	T = 3.59	p = <0.0001

As illustrated in Table XV, correlation of the right and left USSEP N19 latencies increases with chemical exposure, r = 0.05 and p = <0.85 prior to exposure and r = 0.42 and p = <0.08 during exposure. The correlation of the right and left P22 latencies is r = 0.18 and p = <0.50 before exposure and r = 0.67 and p = <0.0001 during exposure.

Table XVI
Correlation of Right and Left Upper SSEP Amplitude
Prior to and During Chemical Exposure

N19 Amplitude prior to	R = 0.92	T = 9.38	p = <0.0001
N19 Amplitude during	R = 0.05	T = 0.19	p = <0.85
P22 Amplitude prior to	R = 0.86	T = 6.42	p = <0.0001
P22 Amplitude during	R = 0.10	T = 0.16	p = <0.88

As illustrated in Table XVI, correlation of the right and left amplitudes of USSEP N19 decreases with exposure to chemical, from r = 0.92 and p = <0.0001 before exposure to r = 0.05 and p = <0.85 after. The correlation of the right and left P22 amplitudes also decreases with exposure to chemical, from r = 0.86 and p = <0.0001 to r = 0.10 and p = <0.88.

Table XVII
Correlation of Right and Left Lower SSEP Latency
Prior to and During Chemical Exposure

P37 Latency prior to	R = 0.49	T = 2.25	p = <0.04
P37 Latency during	R = 0.79	T = 5.11	p = <0.0001
N45 Latency prior to	R = 0.48	T = 2.17	p = <0.05
N45 Latency during	R = 0.76	T = 4.63	p = <0.0001

As illustrated in Table XVII, correlation of the right and left LSSEP P37 latencies increases during exposure, from r = 0.49 and p = <0.04 before exposure to r = 0.79 and p = <0.0001 after. Right and left N45 correlation of latencies also increased during exposure from r = 0.48 and p = <0.05 to r = 0.76 and p = <0.0001.

Table XVIII
Correlation of Right and Left Lower SSEP Amplitude
Prior to and During Chemical Exposure

P37 Amplitude prior to	R = 0.91	T = 8.83	p = <0.0001
P37 Amplitude during	R = 0.04	T = 0.16	p = <0.88
N45 Amplitude prior to	R = 0.86	T = 6.84	p = <0.0001
N45 Amplitude during	R = 0.01	T = 0.04	p = <0.97

As illustrated in Table XVIII, the right and left LSSEP P37 amplitudes correlate well before exposure and not at all during exposure: r = 0.91

and p = <0.0001 before and r = 0.04 and p = <0.88 after. The right and left LSSEP N45 amplitudes also correlate well before exposure and not at all during exposure: r = 0.86 and p = <0.0001 before and r = 0.01 and p = <0.97 after.

DISCUSSION

This study had one aim: To determine whether the disability reported by MCS patients on exposure to chemicals is associated with similar and measurable changes in brain function. In the 20 patients studied, the association proved obvious. The patients had diffuse, similar and disturbingly severe changes as measured by evoked potentials. In addition, although not reported in this study, the psychophysical measurements of disability were significantly increased with exposure to chemicals. The psychophysical ratings of the patients prior to exposure (at least one week chemically free) ranged from 1 to 10 with a mean of 4 (5 being unable to work). All of the ratings during exposure were between 8 and 10 with a mean of 9. Two patients developed seizures during exposure, which resulted in an automatic 10 (totally incapacitated). The chemical exposure produced significant increases in symptomatology (p = <0.0001) that were consistent with the changes in P300 and the patients' inability to work.

Experience shows us that people without chemical sensitivity generally do not have the same changes in response to these chemicals. Certainly the author and the technician working with these patients did not. Supporting this observation are studies demonstrating the vulnerability of a portion of the population to chemical exposure above and beyond the vulnerability of the general population.[3,16,17]

In addition to the above absolute changes in amplitude and latency, the correlations between the right and left sides before and during chemical exposure may be useful as markers for chemical sensitivity. The auditory and visual P300 latencies showed no correlation between right and left sides prior to chemical exposure and a highly significant correlation during chemical exposure. However, the right and left auditory and visual P300 amplitudes showed a high correlation prior to exposure and a lower but still significant correlation during exposure. These changes in correlation are seen as further evidence of the impact of chemicals on the brain in these 20 patients.

As indicated in the beginning of this chapter, factors creating negative bias towards the olfactory system include attitudes expressed in authoritative medical textbooks since at least 1875; the use of technology better suited to other systems (e.g., the immune system) to study the olfactory system; the lack of adverse effect occurring from ablation of olfactory tracts in the brain (which has been misinterpreted as evidence that the system must have little value); the supposed failure to identify neurotransmitters in the olfactory system; and the supposed failure to identify any essential role this system could have in disease production. To varying degrees, these factors influence the attitudes of both professionals and nonprofessionals and generate considerable negativity towards MCS patients who point to olfaction as the major source of their medical problems. Both professionals and nonprofessionals tend to believe that these patients have psychiatric disorders or are simply malingering — a belief that is inconsistent with the data presented in this study, and a belief that has no business in science.

An issue of major importance, from this author's point of view, is the fact that neurotransmitters have been found for the olfactory system, and that many are excitatory amino acids such as glutamate and NMDA, or precursors to excitatory amino acids. These are the same amino acids that are implicated in brain-cell injury and death. They are related to such problems as stroke, pain, depression, and degenerative brain disease.[18]

Glutamate, NMDA, and other excitatory amino acids injure cells when released. This injury makes the cell vulnerable to the influx of chloride ions and then to the influx of calcium ions.[19,20] A fanciful way of looking at this process is to imagine a balloon being inflated until it bursts. It is postulated that olfactory signals release excitatory amino acids, which lead to cell injury that proceeds to the above process. If such a mechanism is in operation, it should be possible to produce the symptoms of MCS by using excitatory amino acid agonists, and to decrease them by using antagonists. The agonists are the volatile short-chain carbon fragments such as formaldehyde, acetone, and methyl-ethyl ketone. Molecules such as these, with the same or fewer carbon units than glutamate, can be agonists. These compounds lead to the release of excitatory amino acids that begin destruction of brain tissue.[21]

In general, odor thresholds decline with exposure to chemicals having more than six carbon fragments and increase with exposure to chemicals having six or fewer carbon fragments.[22] The optimal carbon length for producing excitatory amino acid release is six or fewer. It needs to be emphasized that it is not the carbon chain length of the parent compound that counts. It is the carbon chain length of the volatile component. In other words, analyzing carpet adhesive is of little use; the volatile fragment from carpet adhesive needs to be analyzed.

On the other hand, compounds with greater than six carbon fragments, with a D-configuration and certain other characteristics, can be antagonists of excitatory amino acids.[21,23] These compounds, such as MK801 and dextromethorphan hydrobromide, should decrease symptoms of patients with MCS if the hypothesis is correct. Dextromethorphan hydrobromide, a known excitatory amino acid blocker, does significantly decrease symptoms on olfactory exposure to volatile short-chain carbon compounds in MCS patients. It has been used by the author in more than 30 of these patients with significant positive effect. Dextromethorphan hydrobromide has a remarkable track record and has been used in billions of doses as a cough suppressant without significant biologic problems. To the author's knowledge MK801, an experimental amino acid blocker, has not been used in patients with MCS.

Of considerable importance to the influence of the olfactory system on other parts of the brain is the fact that some signals from the receptor cells and the olfactory bulb are sent to other parts of the brain without modulating nerve centers. Also, in the olfactory bulb approximately 15,000 receptor axons from olfactory receptors in the nose connect with one primary mitral cell. This is the third and perhaps not the final level of augmentation of signal. From the olfactory bulb signals are sent out to nearly every part of the brain. In the present study it was demonstrated that the effect of the olfactory system on the auditory and visual systems is substantial. Thus a receptor system covering about two square centimeters and having only 6 million ciliated receptor cells has an unsuspected disproportionate influence.[24]

The olfactory system produces evoked potentials in the same manner as that observed in the auditory and visual systems. The cerebral generator is in the region where the central sulcus and the sylvian fissure merge. This region is also closely related to pain, emotion, and cognition; thus olfaction may, in some way, relate to MCS patients' problems in these areas. (A review of the pathways leading to and from the olfactory system is provided by Serby and Chobar. Of particular interest are chapters 5 and 6.[25,26]) Lastly, it should be noted that the findings in this study are consistent with a recent SPECT brain scan study by Callender.[27]

SUMMARY

Information was presented demonstrating that olfactory stimulation with chemicals having six or fewer carbon fragments has significant influence on the auditory and visual P300. Left and right auditory and visual P300 latencies were prolonged to a highly significant degree following olfactory stimulation. Both right and left auditory P300 amplitudes were significantly decreased. The visual P300 amplitude was not significantly changed during stimulation, but the quality of the waveform was changed, and two patients developed occipital seizures. There were also statistically significant increases in psychophysical measurements of disability and symptoms. Since olfactory signals are sent to almost every part of the brain, it is possible that this system's use of excitatory amino acids in neurotransmission could lead to brain-cell injury and subsequent neuronal changes that are experienced as the signs and symptoms of MCS.

This paper was presented to the Society for Neurosciences, 24th Annual Meeting, Miami, Florida, 1994; and to the Center for Disease Control Seminar on the Chemical Impact Project, National Center for Environmental Health, Atlanta, Georgia, 1995. It was abstracted in *Society for Neuroscience Abstracts* **20** (1994); 606.10.

References

1. Goodin, D. S., and M. J. Aminoff: "Evaluation of dementia by event-related potentials." *J Clin Neurophysiol,* 1992; 9: 521–525.
2. Terr, A. I.: "Multiple chemical sensitivities." *Immunology and Allergy Clinics of North America,* 1993; 12: 897–908.
3. Bell, I. R., C. S. Miller, and G. E. Schwartz: "An olfactory-limbic model of multiple chemical sensitivity syndrome: possible relationships to kindling and affective spectrum disorders." *Biol Psychiatry,* 1992; 32: 218–242.
4. Dalton, J. C.: *A Treatise on Human Physiology,* 4th edition (Philadelphia: Lea, 1876), 430.
5. Brodal, A.: *Neurological Anatomy in Relation to Clinical Medicine,* 3d edition (New York and Oxford: Oxford University Press, 1981), 640–697.
6. Greer, C. A.: "Structural organization of the olfactory system." Chap. 4 in T. V. Getchell, R. L. Doty, L. M. Bartoshuk, and J. B. Snow, Jr. (eds.), *Smell and Taste in Health and Disease* (New York: Raven, 1991), 65, 76, 77.
7. Picton, T. M.: "The P300 wave of the human event-related potential," *J Clin Neurophysiol,* 1992; 9: 456–479.
8. Cullen, M. R.: "The worker with multiple chemical sensitivities: an overview," *Occupational Medicine,* 1987; 2: 655–661.
9. Stevens, S. L.: "The psychophysical law" and "Sensation and measurement."

Chaps. 1 and 2 in S. L. Stevens, *Psychophysics: Introduction to Its Perceptual, Neural and Social Prospects* (New York: Wiley, 1975), 1–62.

10. Olverman, J. J., and J. C. Watkins: "NMDA agonists and antagonists." Chap. 2 in J. C. Watkins and G. L. Collingridge (eds.), *The NMDA Receptor* (Oxford, New York, and Tokyo: IRL Press at Oxford University Press, 1989), 30–34.

11. *Cadwell Laboratories Manual, Cadwell Spectrum 32* (Kennewick, Wash.: Cadwell World Laboratories, 1993), 31–1 to 40–2.

12. Pritchard, W. S.: "Psychophysiology of P300," *Psychological Bulletin,* 1989; 89: 506–540.

13. Ullsperger, P., H. G. Gille, and A. M. Metkz: "The P300 as a metric in psychophysics of cognitive potentials." Chap. 48 in C. Barber and T. Blum (eds.), *Evoked Potentials III: The Third International Evoked Potentials Symposium* (Boston and London: Butterworth, 1987), 355–360.

14. Patterson, J. V. , H. J. Michalewski, and A. Starr: "Latency variability of the components of auditory event-related potentials to infrequent stimuli in aging, Alzheimer-type dementia and depression," *Electroen and Clin Neurophys,* 1988; 71; 450–460.

15. Glantz, S. A.: *Primer of Biostatistics* [computer program] (New York: McGraw-Hill, Health Professionals Div., 1992).

16. Bell, I. R., G. E. Schwartz, J. M. Peterson, D. Amend, and W. A. Stini: "Possible time-dependent sensitization to xenobiotics: self-reported illness from chemical odors, foods, and opiate drugs in an older population," *Arch Environ Health,* 1993; 48: 315–327.

17. Wilcox, P. P.: "Impaired erythrocyte pyruvate kinase activity in chemical sensitivity syndrome." Paper accepted for presentation to the Society of Toxicology Annual Meeting, Dallas, Tex., March 1994.

18. Garthwaite, G.: "NMDA receptors, neural development and neural degeneration." Chap. 14 in J. C. Watkins and G. L. Collingridge (eds.), *The NMDA Receptor* (Oxford, New York, and Tokyo: IRL Press at Oxford University Press, 1989), 187–205.

19. Iverson, L. L., G. N. Woodruff, J. A. Kemp, A. C. Foster, R. Gill, and E. H. F. Wong: "Pharmacology and neuroprotective effects of the NMDA antagonist MK801," in E. F. Domino and J. M. Kamenka (eds.), *Sigma and Phencyclidine-like Compounds as Molecular Probes in Biology* (Ann Arbor, Mich.: NPP, 1988), 757–766.

20. Marcoux, F. W., J. E. Goodrick, A. W. Probert, Jr., and M. A. Dominick: "Ketamine prevents glutamate-induced calcium influx and ischemic nerve cell injury," in E. F. Domino and J. M. Kamenka (eds.), *Sigma and Phencyclidine-like Compounds as Molecular Probes in Biology* (Ann Arbor, Mich: NPP, 1988), 735–748.

21. Iverson, L. L., G. N. Woodruff, J. A. Kemp, A. C. Foster, R. McKernan, and E. H. F. Wong: "Non-competitive NMDA antagonists as drugs." Chap. 16 in J. C. Watkins and G. L. Collingridge (eds.), *The NMDA Receptor* (Oxford, New York, and Tokyo: IRL Press at Oxford University Press, 1989), 217–226.

22. Cometto-Muniz, J. E., and W. E. Cain: "Influence of airborne contaminants on olfaction and common chemical sense." Chap. 49 in T. V. Getchell, R. L. Doty, L. M. Bartoshuk, and J. B. Snow, Jr. (eds.), *Smell and Taste in Health and Disease* (New York: Raven, 1991), 765–785.

23. Meldrum, B. S., A. G. Chapman, S. Patel, and J. Swan: "Competitive NMDA agonists as drugs." Chap. 15 in J. C. Watkins and G. L. Collingridge (eds.), *The NMDA Receptor* (Oxford, New York, and Tokyo: IRL Press at Oxford University Press, 1989), 207–216.

24. Kinnamon, S. C., and T. V. Getchell: "Sensory transduction in olfactory recep-

tor neurons and gustatory receptor cells." Chap. 9 in T. V. Getchell, R. L. Doty, L. M. Bartoshuk, and J. B. Snow, Jr. (eds.), *Smell and Taste in Health and Disease* (New York: Raven, 1991), 145–172.

25. McClean, J. H., and M. T. Shipley: "Neuroanatomical substrate of olfaction." Chap. 5 in J. J. Serby and K. L. Chobar (eds.), *Science of Olfaction* (New York: Springer-Verlag, 1992), 126–171.

26. Nickell, W. T., and M. T. Shipley: "Neurophysiology of the olfactory bulb." Chap. 6 in J. J. Serby and K. L. Chobar (eds.), *Science of Olfaction* (New York: Springer-Verlag, 1992), 172–212.

27. Callender, T. J., L. Morrow, K. Subramanian, D. Duhon, and M. Ristovv: "Three-dimensional brain metabolic imaging in patients with toxic encephalopathy." *Environmental Research,* 1993; 60: 295–319.

3. SPECT BRAIN SCANNING AFTER CHEMICAL INJURY

Gunnar Heuser, M.D., Ph.D., F.A.C.P.

Acknowledgment: *All SPECT scans referred to in this article were performed under the supervision of Dr. Ismael Mena at Harbor-UCLA and were interpreted by him. The author of this chapter then reinterpreted Dr. Mena's report in the context of the clinical history and other findings on each patient. In view of this cooperative effort, this article is narrated in the first person plural ("we" and "our"), referring to Dr. Mena and the author.*

While certain public interest and government agencies promote the awareness of the potential cancer-causing effects of chemicals, awareness of the potential neurotoxic effects has remained very limited. Yet these neurotoxic effects may be with us presently and may affect the intellectual performance and emotional stability of our children, and of the adolescent, adult, and elderly populations. Increasing awareness of the potential significance of neurotoxic exposure is expressed in a number of recent publications.

Potentially neurotoxic exposure is frequent in our society. Intermittent contact with solvents and pesticides is an almost daily occurrence. Neurotoxic chemicals are found in our work environment (e.g. solvents), home environment (e.g. some carpets and paints), tap water and imported dinnerware (which may contain lead), and commuting environment (gasoline, diesel, products of combustion), and can originate from some hobbies (e.g. photo developers, oil paints). In addition, we may knowingly or unknowingly encounter pesticides and other chemicals at work, at home, in foods and while traveling. Superimposed on these everyday exposures may be a more significant incidental or accidental exposure.

[27]

Both symptoms and objective abnormalities arising from *acute* exposure to potentially neurotoxic chemicals are well described in the literature. Information on acute exposure is easily found in textbooks and also easily available from poison control centers. It is generally assumed that patients will fully recover from the effects of acute exposure.

The literature regarding the potentially *delayed* or long-lasting effects of neurotoxic exposure is sparse by comparison. This lack of solid data is in part explained by the fact that sophisticated methodology to study late neurotoxic effects was not available or not used in the past.

In recent years, SPECT brain imaging has shown its usefulness in many clinical settings and has now become an acknowledged diagnostic tool in patients with a variety of central nervous system diseases. It has also become an acknowledged diagnostic tool in the study of toxic exposure. Finally, SPECT is now discussed as a diagnostic tool in some textbooks on neurotoxicology, and toxic exposure is mentioned in some texts on SPECT.

Many researchers have used either xenon (radioactive gas by inhalation) or HMPAO (radioactive compound given intravenously) in their studies. We believe that both are helpful since they complement each other. Xenon studies show global and regional cerebral blood flow in absolute measurements. HMPAO studies show relative distribution of blood flow (perfusion) and also depend in part on the permeability of the blood-brain barrier and intracompartmental distribution and metabolism in the brain.

SPECT scans are frequently evaluated by one or two readers who decide whether they are abnormal. This approach is less than satisfactory since statements regarding abnormalities are then based solely on visual inspection and not on comparisons with normal controls.

Our interpretation of SPECT scans is based on comparisons with a normal population (age-matched controls). This method makes it possible to make statistically valid statements regarding abnormalities.

In 1992 we suggested the use of SPECT as a sensitive indicator of central nervous system impairment after neurotoxic exposure. In 1993 Callender et al. reported that a series of patients had shown abnormal SPECT after occupational neurotoxic exposure.

While some researchers have chosen PET scanning or P300 evoked response studies as their diagnostic tools to assess toxic exposure, we have continued to explore SPECT.

Our studies show that significant impairment of cerebral perfusion (blood flow with oxygen delivery) can be seen in the frontal, temporal, and parietal lobes after neurotoxic chemical exposure and that this impairment may continue for years thereafter. This impairment correlates clinically with continuing complaints of neurocognitive dysfunction.

Hypoperfusion is asymmetrical in distribution in many cases. While any given individual case may show predominantly left- or right-sided impairment, our young patient population shows predominantly left-sided impairment while the elderly show predominantly right-sided hypoperfusion (HMPAO).

Our preliminary data show that a mathematical task will "light up" certain areas of a normal brain on SPECT. This activation is frequently absent in patients with neurocognitive impairment after neurotoxic exposure.

Our preliminary data also show that a patient with MCS will demonstrate further impairment of the SPECT brain scan when exposed to a small amount of some perfumes.

Most of our patients unfortunately did not show evidence of recovery, especially of neuropsychological function.

In my clincal practice, I do not see patients during and immediately after toxic exposure. Instead, I see patients who do not feel that they have recovered and therefore request objective documentation of their problems. Since we have not had the opportunity to compare these patients with a larger population of exposed patients, we are unable at this time to estimate what percentage of exposed patients eventually develop chronic impairment. This still needs to be studied.

The type of SPECT abnormality seen after toxic exposure does not at this time allow us to draw any conclusions about how time of exposure (recent or years ago) and type of exposure (pesticide vs. solvent vs. other chemicals) relate to abnormality.

While our data did not show any difference between groups of chemicals, it is important to note that careful analysis of a given exposure usually reveals the involvement of more than one chemical. "Toxic" carpet and related materials contain a multitude of potentially toxic chemicals, some or all of which may be detrimental to a patient's health. Pesticides always contain "inert" materials and often propellants and contaminants which may be more toxic than the material noted on the label. Furthermore, multiple chemicals may interact with each other before and after entry into the organism. They may also interact with chemicals already present in the environment or may be transformed to other chemicals when exposed to heat. All these factors have to be considered. It is easy to see why one chemical can rarely be measured and pinpointed as the cause of toxic effects.

[29]

The cause of hypoperfusion is not known at this time. Cellular (neuronal) damage with down-regulation of cerebral blood flow, damage to blood vessels, and finally atrophy of the cerebral cortex all have to be considered. Vasculitis seems less likely since some of our patients showed temporary normalization of perfusion after intravenous Diamox. It seems more likely that the affected brain cells cannot be properly activated and cannot "call for" more blood supply and oxygen to support their increased activity.

Most of our patients had had nondiagnostic MRI brain scans. Therefore, significant cell death was not a feature in our patient population. Nevertheless, the population suffered severe functional impairment, found not only on SPECT brain scanning but also when patients were tested by a neuropsychologist.

Not all patients in the same toxic environment will suffer the same effects. Women and children are more often affected than adult males. In addition to sex and age, genetic predisposition seems to be a major determinant in susceptibility to toxic exposure. Currently no commercially available tests can investigate genetic predisposition in meaningful detail.

In conclusion, we found mostly asymmetrical impairment of perfusion in our patients after neurotoxic exposure. In more severely affected patients we also found random impairment of perfusion throughout the cerebral cortex in a scalloping pattern. This impairment was in our opinion severe enough in some patients to account for significant abnormalities on neuropsychological testing as well as abnormalities in behavior.

References

Callender, T. J., L. Morrow, K. Subramanian, D. Duhon, and M. Ristovv: "Three-dimensional brain metabolic imaging in patients with toxic encephalopathy." *Environmental Research*, 1993; 60: 295–319.

Fincher, C. E., T. Chang, E. Harrell, et al.: "Comparison of single photon emission computed tomography findings in cases of healthy adults and solvent-exposed adults." *American Journal of Industrial Medicine*, 1997; 31: 4–14.

Heuser, G.: "Editorial: diagnostic markers in clinical immunotoxicology and neurotoxicology." *Journal of Occupational Medicine and Toxicology*, 1992; 1 (4): v.

Heuser, G., I. Mena, and F. Alamos: Neurospect findings in patients exposed to neurotoxic chemicals." *Toxicology and Industrial Health*, 1994; 10 (4/5): 561–571.

Heuser, G., A. Vodjani, and S. Heuser: "Diagnostic markers of multiple chemical sensitivity." In *Multiple Chemical Sensitivities*, by the Board on Environmental Studies and Toxicology, Commission on Life Sciences, National Research Council. Washington, D.C.: National Academy Press, 1992.

Van Heertum, R. L., and R. S. Tikofsky, eds.: *Cerebral SPECT Imaging*. New York: Raven, 1995.

4. PORPHYRIA, CYTOCHROME P-450, AND TOXIC EXPOSURE

Bonnye L. Matthews

In the field of MCS, perhaps the most significant finding in recent years is that many chemical sensitives have a recognized disease known as porphyria. Though doctors have long been acquainted with porphyria, it was previously thought to be only an inherited condition, and very rare. To get an idea of how rare, consider that a liver specialist might see six cases in a lifetime of practice.

Studies have demonstrated that in genetically predisposed individuals, porphyria can be touched off by certain chemicals. Now, evidence suggests that some chemicals can induce porphyria in people who are *not* genetically predisposed. Doctors are finding that up to 90 percent of their MCS patients show positive results on tests for porphyria.

The porphyria connection has done much to clarify the mechanics of MCS, but it hasn't done anything to make MCS visible to the casual observer. Porphyria is not like a broken leg, a health problem that is obvious at a glance and easy to understand. Porphyria is both invisible and terribly complex. Nevertheless, it is worth the effort of explaining, since with understanding of porphyria it is now possible, for the first time, to create a model of MCS. This model at least makes the disorder visible on paper, no matter how persistently it remains concealed in the sufferer.

SOME IMPORTANT DEFINITIONS

According to *Harrison's Principles of Internal Medicine,* 13th edition, "porphyrias are inherited or acquired disorders of specific enzymes in the heme biosynthetic pathway."[28] More precisely, these disorders are *deficits* of certain enzymes; that is, the enzymes are present in subnormal or insufficient quantities. In case this definition sounds like a lot of words and not much communication, here are some further definitions that may be useful:

- *Enzymes* are complex proteins that cause changes in other substances, though they themselves do not change.
- A *biosynthetic pathway* is a metabolic process that generates a product.
- *Metabolic processes* are the body's way of taking in food, water, and oxygen and changing them to substances required for growth and maturity, mechanical energy, and heat.
- The *heme biosynthetic pathway* is the metabolic process for producing heme.
- *Heme* is an iron-containing pigment that combines with other substances to produce *hemoproteins,* such as *hemoglobin* (which enables red blood cells to transport oxygen) and *cytochromes* (also involved in oxidation as well as other tasks).

These definitions make it clear that porphyrias are deficiencies of specific enzymes required for the production of heme. Such disorders can cause cells to build up damaging levels of porphyrins or in some cases decrease the production of hemoproteins. A decrease in hemoproteins could have a neurologic effect.

A few more definitions are necessary. We have observed that enzymes cause changes in certain other substances with which they come in contact. It may be helpful to think of the heme manufacturing process as an assembly line, and enzymes as workers along that line, producing specific changes in the materials that pass by. Now we need some names for those materials.

The heme manufacturing process begins with a substance called *delta-*

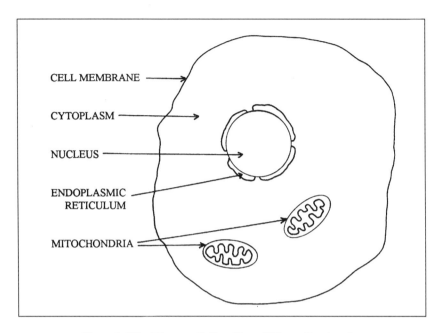

CELL MEMBRANE

CYTOPLASM

NUCLEUS

ENDOPLASMIC
RETICULUM

MITOCHONDRIA

Chart 1. The Human Cell — Site of Heme Production

aminolevulinic acid formed from succinyl coenzyme A at the end of the
Krebs cycle combined with glycine and acted on by the enzyme delta
aminolevulinic synthase. Because delta-aminolevulinic acid is the first material — a predecessor or "ancestor" to substances yet to be formed — it is classified as a *precursor*. Its first contact with an enzyme (delta-aminolevulinate
dehydratase) produces yet another precursor, called *porphobilinogen*.

Now the process begins to transform precursors into substances called
porphyrins. These are nitrogen-containing chemicals that are necessary
to respiration. As porphyrins pass along the heme biosynthetic pathway,
they interact with a number of enzymes to produce still other porphyrins.
Some of these porphyrins are excreted; others continue along the pathway
and ultimately contribute to the production of heme and hemoproteins.

The production of heme occurs in most cells of the human body, but
especially in the liver cells, blood cells, skin cells, and nerve cells. Chart 1
illustrates the basic heme-producing structure' of the cell.

The cell consists of a cell membrane filled with a fluid called cytoplasm, which contains various structures. Some of those structures are
the cell nucleus (the "brains" of the cell, where DNA is kept and RNA

transcribed); the mitochondria (sites of aerobic respiration for energy production); and the endoplasmic reticulum (site of modification or storage of certain molecules). The parts of the cell specifically related to the manufacture of heme are the cytoplasm and the mitochondria.

The processes of metabolism related to porphyria are as follows:

1. *Glycolysis,* in which glucose is broken down to water, carbon, and adenosine triphosphate (ATP). ATP is a molecule that stores energy like a battery and releases it when needed. (See Chart 2.)
2. *Formation of acetyl coenzyme A* (acetyl CoA). (See Chart 2.)
3. The Krebs cycle, by which succinyl CoA is formed. (See Chart 2.)
4. *Heme synthesis,* in which hemoproteins are produced. Hemoproteins include heme, the cytochromes including cytochrome P-450, and others. At points along the heme synthesis pathway, depending on the point, various types of porphyria may result from enzyme deficits. (See Chart 3.)

On Chart 3 porphyrins are identified in bold face type. They are further identified as a name followed by a number. Enzymes are identified by italic type. When experts are discussing porphyria they speak of precursors, porphyrins and enzymes. Just to sort these out for clarity they are:

Precursors	Porphyrins	Enzymes
delta-aminolevulinic acid	uroporphyrinogen I	porphobilinogen deaminase
porphobilinogen	heptacarboxylporphyrinogen I	uroporphyrinogen decarboxylase
	hexacarboxylporphyrinogen I	uroporphyrinogen III synthase
	pentacarboxylporphyrinogen I	coproporphyrinogen oxidase
	coproporphyrinogen I	protoporphyrinogen oxidase
	uroporphryrinogen III	ferrochelatase
	heptacarboxylporphyrinogen III	
	hexacarboxylporphyrinogen III	
	pentacarboxylporphyrinogen III	
	coproporphyrinogen III	
	tricarboxylporphyrinogen III	
	protoporphyrinogen IX	
	protoporphyrin IX	

Fuel Source:
food broken down to sugar

Process 1: GLYCOLYSIS (Glycolysis means splitting sugar. This process occurs in the cytoplasm of cells and bacteria)

Glycolysis is the initial sequence used by cells to break down sugars. ATP is both required to initiate the process and is an outcome of it. ATP is made of adenine, ribose, and a tail made of phosphates. Adding a phosphate requires energy; releasing one provides energy. ATP can be viewed as a battery, storing energy when it is not needed, releasing it when it is needed.

Aerobic Glycolysis (This process takes food and oxygen to produce energy and carbon dioxide and water):
$$C_6H_{12}O_6 + 6O_2 + 36ADP + 36Pi \text{--------} > 6CO_2 + 6H_2O + 36ATP$$
$$\text{carbon} \quad \text{water} \quad \text{adenosine triphosphate}$$

Anaerobic Glycolysis (This process consists of 9 steps and requires no gaseous oxygen to effect the breakdown):
Step 1. A molecule of ATP breaks down and forms ADP + **glucose-6-phosphate**
Step 2. Glucose-6-phosphate becomes **fructose-6-phosphate**
Step 3. A molecule of ATP breaks down and a phosphate is added to fructose-6-phosphate to make **fructose-1, 6-diphosphate**
Step 4. Fructose-1, 6-diphosphate breaks down into 2 3-carbon molecules: **phosphoglyceraldehyde (PGAL)**
Step 5. PGAL oxidizes as NAD^+ (nicotine adenine dinucleotide), accepting 2 electrons to become **NADH**. PGAL reacts with free phosphate in the cell to yield **1, 3 diphosphoglycerate (DPGA)**
Step 6. Each DPGA molecule loses one phosphate group and goes to an ADP molecule to yield **2 ATP** and 2 3-phosphoglycerate molecules (**3-PGA**)
Step 7. 3-PGA is converted to **2-PGA**
Step 8. Both 2-PGA molecules lose water and become **2 phosphoenol pyruvate molecules (PEP)**
Step 9. PEP gives a phosphate to ADP which results in **ATP** and **pyruvate**

Process Yield: 2 NADH molecules, **2 ATP** molecules, **2 pyruvate** molecules

Process 2: FORMATION OF ACETYL COENZYME A (pyruvic molecules are transported to the mitochondria where the remainder of this transformation occurs)

$$2 \text{ pyruvate} + 2 \text{ } NAD^+ + 2 \text{ CoA} \text{ ------} > \textbf{2 acetyl CoA} + \textbf{2 NADH} + \textbf{carbon dioxide}$$

Process 3: THE KREBS CYCLE (Also called the tricarboxylic acid cycle and citric acid cycle. This cycle occurs in the mitochondria.)

This process begins with pyruvic acid from glycolysis combined with products from the fatty acid cycle to form acetyl coenzyme A. This metabolic process breaks down carbohydrates, proteins, and fats. Here the process is highly oversimplified. Acetyl coenzyme A changes to citric acid which changes to cis-aconitic acid which changes to isocitric acid which changes to oxalosuccinic acid which changes to fumaric acid which changes to malic acid which changes to oxaloacetic acid, and then the cycle repeats. Just before succinate acid is formed, succinyl coenzyme A is produced. Succinyl coenzyme A is the beginning of the metabolic process for heme and the focus of porphyria.

$$\text{oxaloacetate} + \text{acetyl CoA} + 2H_2O + ADP + Pi + 3NAD^+ + FAD \text{--------} >$$

$$\textbf{oxaloacetate} + \textbf{2}CO_2 + \textbf{CoA} + \textbf{ATP} + \textbf{3NAHD} + \textbf{3H+} + \textbf{FADH}_2$$

Products from this cycle also include:
malic acid, succinic acid, fumaric acid, and (**succinyl CoA**)

Chart 2. Human Metabolism to Produce Succinyl Coenzyme A

Process 4: HEME SYNTHESIS (This process occurs partly in the mitochondria and partly in the cytoplasm.)

The major sites of hemoproteins are in tissue that pertains to red blood cells: polychromatic erythroblasts, reticulocytes, and nucleated erythrocytes in bone marrow. Hemoproteins are all involved in some way with oxygen or with oxidative processes. Examples of hemoproteins are: hemoglobin, cytochromes, catalase, perioxidase, and tryptophan oxygenase.

Note: In the chart below, names appearing in boldface type are porphyrins. Names in italics are enzymes.

MITOCHONDRIA

heme and other hemoproteins

cofactor vitamin B-6+　succinyl CoA　　　+　　　glycine
　　　　　　　　　　　(from Krebs cycle)　　　(from general amino acid pool)

ferrochelatase
protoporphyrin IX
protoporphyrinogen oxidase
protoporphyrinogen IX

delta-aminolevulinate synthase　　　　　　*coproporphyrinogen oxidase*
tricarboxylporphyrinogen III
coproporphyrinogen oxidase

delta-aminolevulinic acid
MITOCHONDRIA　　　　　　　　　　　　　　**coproporphyrinogen III**

- -

CYTOPLASM　　　　delta-aminolevulinic acid　　**coproporphyrinogen III**
uroporphyrinogen decarboxylase
pentacarboxylporphyrinogen III
uroporphyrinogen decarboxylase
delta-aminolevulinate dehydratase　　　　**hexacarboxylporphyrinogen III**
uroporphyrinogen decarboxylase
heptacarboxylporphyrinogen III
uroporphyrinogen decarboxylase

porphobilinogen
porphobilinogen deaminase
hydroxymethylbilane---*uroporphyrinogen*
III synthase--- **uroporphyrinogen III**

uroporphyrinogen I
uroporphyrinogen decarboxylase
heptacarboxylporphyrinogen I
uroporphyrinogen decarboxylase
hexacarboxylporphyrinogen I
uroporphyrinogen decarboxylase
pentacarboxylporphyrinogen I
uroporphyrinogen decarboxylase
coproporphyrinogen I ————— excreted in urine and bile
CYTOPLASM

Chart 3. Human Metabolism to Produce Heme

Note that the porphyrins start with a name and end with a number. The porphyrins that end with I are excreted; their function is unknown.

Now, let us lay the processes outlined in Charts 2 and 3 over the illustration of the cell. (See Chart 4.) This arrangement makes the production of heme more visible.

Charts 2, 3, and 4 depict the normal functioning of the heme biosynthetic pathway. Remember, porphyria is an *abnormal* state involving deficiencies of specific enzymes along the way.

The first sign of abnormality is an overabundance of precursors and porphyrins. Let us return for a moment to our assembly line metaphor.

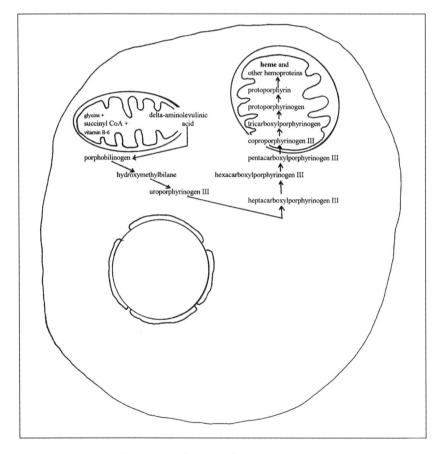

Chart 4. Production of Heme in the Cell

Workstations along the line are the sites of porphyrin metabolism (the points at which porphyrins are transformed into new porphyrins). What happens if a worker (an enzyme) is missing from a workstation? Work piles up. Instead of being metabolized, certain porphyrins accumulate. In a factory, they'd be spilling off the conveyor belt and onto the floor — a fanciful image, but not inaccurate for our purposes.

PORPHYRINOPATHIES

Porphyrin metabolism may be disordered in several ways, not all of which can be classified as porphyrias. Some are *porphyrinopathies*. Porphyrinopathies are obvious disorders but are not characterized by an enzyme deficit as are porphyrias.

Porphyrinuria. In a huge study being conducted by the Superfund Basic Research Program, a group of federal agencies and universities across the country are studying, among other things, toxic event–related biomarkers. This information is available on the internet at the following address:

http://www.niehs.nih.gov/sbrp/newweb/sftext01.htm.

Their research has included porphyrinuria (porphyrins in urine) as a biomarker. A biomarker identifies toxic exposure, not disease. The research, for example, has identified porphyrins in the urine of dentists who have been inserting amalgam fillings. Dentists may show porphyrinuria in a nondisease state.

Precursor-porphyrinuria. Porphyrinogenic substances (things that cause disorders in porphyrin synthesis) can provoke overproduction of precursors along with porphyrins in the presence of diminished enzymes. The quantity depends upon the amount of exposure to porphyrinogenic substances. This *precursor-porphyrinuria* may stop short of active porphyria, or, if the exposure continues, it may generate porphyria. Porphyrinogenic substances can also cause other nonporphyria or preporphyria effects.

Delta-aminolevulinate overproduction. Delta-aminolevulinate is neurotoxic. Delta-aminolevulinate overproduction can produce neurotoxic effects or lead to the production of neuropathic porphyrias. According to Ellefson and Ford (1996), "neuropathic expression occurs in both the central and peripheral neural systems and affects sensory, motor, autonomic, and mental functions" (page S120).

PORPHYRIAS

What separates porphyria from other disorders of porphyrin metabolism is the demonstrated deficiency of at least one enzyme along the pathway. According to *Harrison's*,[28] "a definite diagnosis requires demonstration of the specific enzyme deficiency" (page 2073). Furthermore, accurate diagnosis requires one additional element: symptoms. Symptoms and signs plus positive test data are the keys to diagnosis. Test data are also required to distinguish between those porphyrias that are inherited, and those that are produced by toxic exposure.

Inherited Porphyria. Inherited porphyria is a genetic disorder. It can show up at birth or later in life. An adult may have a latent condition that remains silent until something sets it off. Inherited porphyrias are associated with specific low enzymes, as follows:

Porphyria Type	Enzyme Deficiency
aminolevulinic dehydratase deficiency	aminolevulinic dehydratase
acute intermittent porphyria	porphobilinogen deaminase
congenital erythropoietic porphyria	uroporphyrinogen III synthase
porphyria cutanea tarda	uroporphyrinogen decarboxylase
coproporphyria	coproporphyrinogen oxidase
variegate porphyria	protoporphyrinogen oxidase
erythropoietic protoporphyria	ferrochelatase

Generally, an individual inherits only one enzyme deficiency and thus only one specific porphyria. Enzyme levels, once established, remain fairly constant.

These porphyrias are categorized as either hepatic (related to the liver) or erythropoietic (related to the production of red blood cells). The category is determined by the site of overproduction and what is overproduced. Depending on the type, porphyrias produce either neurovisceral symptoms or photosensitivity — or, in two cases, both, as shown below.

Porphyria	Enzyme Deficiency	Symptoms
----------------------------	*Hepatic Porphyrias*	----------------------------
aminolevulinic dehydratase deficiency porphyria	delta-aminolevulinic dehydratase	neurovisceral symptoms
acute intermittent porphyria	porphobilinogen deaminase	neurovisceral symptoms
porphyria cutanea tarda	uroporphyrinogen decarboxylase	photosensitivity
coproporphyria	coproporphyrinogen oxidase	neurovisceral symptoms and photosensitivity
variegate porphyria	protoporphyrinogen oxidase	neurovisceral symptoms and photosensitivity
------------------------	*Erythropoietic Porphyrias*	--------------------------
congenital erythropoietic porphyria	uroporphyrinogen III synthase	photosensitivity
erythropoietic protoporphyria	ferrochelatase	photosensitivity

Neurovisceral means that symptoms relate both to the central nervous system and the internal organs. Neurovisceral symptoms include severe abdominal pain, vomiting, constipation, personality changes, paresthesias (numbness or tingling), weakness, paralysis, muscle pain, and dark or red urine. In acute attacks, life-threatening situations may occur, with electrolyte imbalances, low blood pressure, and shock. Photosensitivity is abnormal sensitivity to sunlight; exposure to sunlight produces pain, reddening, blistering, and edema, followed by scarring of skin.

Toxic-Induced Porphyria. Toxic-induced porphyria is acquired through contact with toxic substances that set off a disorder in an otherwise genetically porphyria-free individual. Toxic-induced porphyrias differ from inherited porphyrias in at least two important ways. By strictly avoiding porphyrinogenic substances, people with toxic-induced porphyria may sometimes return their test results to normal (which would be abnormal in inherited porphyrias). However, many experience new development of disease as soon as recontact with porphyrinogenic substances occurs. The number of porphyrinogenic substances exceeds 3,000. Porphyria may be provoked by any one of them. The significance of these facts has not been lost on MCS sufferers. Many individuals with symptoms fitting the symptom complex known as MCS have realized that something set off the

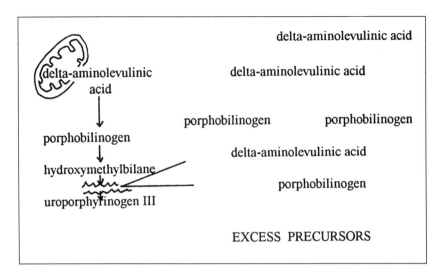

Chart 5. Diminished Uroporphyrinogen III Synthase: Acute Intermittent Porphyria

problem. Later they discovered they were having the same reactions to other chemical exposures. In MCS circles this is called the spreading effect. For those individuals with MCS, finding that they have toxic-induced porphyria gives new meaning to their experience with the spreading effect.

Another difference between inherited and toxic-induced porphyrias is that the inherited variety is virtually always limited to one enzyme deficiency, and the level of the deficient enzyme tends to remain fairly stable. Finding persons with multiple enzyme defects is almost unheard of in inherited porphyrias. In toxic-induced porphyrias it is quite common, and the levels and numbers of enzymes affected vary with exposure.

Whether toxic-induced or inherited, however, porphyrias in their active phases produce the same effects in the sufferer.

Since the metabolic process is not unlike a production line it is possible to visualize porphyria. Chart 5 shows a case of acute intermittent porphyria, in which the diminished enzyme is uroporphyrinogen III synthase (also called porphobilinogen deaminase). The enzyme is operating at 50 percent of normal.

Chart 5 shows that acute intermittent porphyria involves the accumulation of delta-aminolevulinic acid and porphobilinogen in the cell's cytoplasm. That excess moves to the blood and is excreted. Acute intermittent

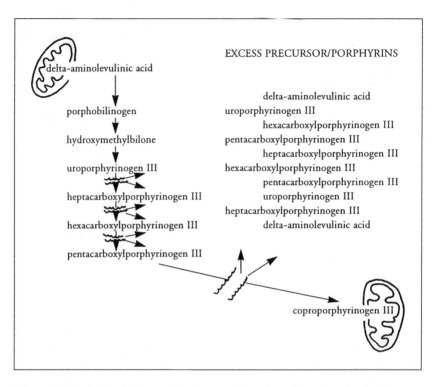

EXCESS PRECURSOR/PORPHYRINS

delta-aminolevulinic acid

porphobilinogen

hydroxymethylbilone

uroporphyrinogen III

heptacarboxylporphyrinogen III

hexacarboxylporphyrinogen III

pentacarboxylporphyrinogen III

delta-aminolevulinic acid
uroporphyrinogen III
hexacarboxylporphyrinogen III
pentacarboxylporphyrinogen III
heptacarboxylporphyrinogen III
hexacarboxylporphyrinogen III
pentacarboxylporphyrinogen III
uroporphyrinogen III
heptacarboxylporphyrinogen III
delta-aminolevulinic acid

coproporphyrinogen III

Chart 6. Diminished Uroporphyrinogen Decarboxylase: Porphyria Cutanea Tarda

porphyria is an hepatic type of porphyria and is characterized by neuro-visceral symptoms. In severe cases respiratory failure can occur.

Chart 6 shows a case of porphyria cutanea tarda, which involves diminished uroporphyrinogen decarboxylase.

Chart 6 illustrates the excessive buildup of porphyrins in porphyria cutanea tarda. The excess porphyrins move to the blood and are excreted. Their presence in skin that is exposed to sunlight can produce the photosensitivity symptoms of redness, blistering, and ultimate scarring.

EXPERIENCING PORPHYRIA

Example of an Hepatic Porphyria Experience. Although individual experience varies, it is possible to describe some common features of a porphyria attack. In acute intermittent porphyria, characterized by neurovisceral symptoms, an attack usually begins with discomfort in the abdomen. The discomfort may feel like enteritis, but enteritis involves inflammation, while this abdominal discomfort is neurologic. The discomfort may be accompanied by nausea. The intensity of abdominal pain varies from uncomfortable to extreme. Constipation and vomiting — or, less frequently, diarrhea — may occur. The abdominal area may swell significantly, putting pressure on the liver. The first few times people experience abdominal swelling, it can cause more concern than the pain in the abdomen. One of the typical comments is, "I'm not pregnant!" The person may, however, look like she is. This swelling can make it difficult to tie shoes, and in some cases it may interfere mildly with breathing. The affected individual may feel that the swelling would go down if only it were possible to urinate, but unfortunately, urination may be very much decreased. Impairment of renal (kidney) function may occur.

In addition to the abdominal symptoms the hepatic experience often involves a rapidly beating heart. This condition, called *tachycardia*, means that the heart is beating at more than 100 beats per minute. This may be accompanied by hypertension (high blood pressure). There is no definitive level for determining what is high blood pressure. As a flexible rule of thumb, if the systolic level is greater than 140 or the diastolic more than 90, then hypertension is probable. For people with low or normal blood pressure, high blood pressure can cause a feeling of being about to explode. Hypertension may be accompanied by tremors and excess sweating. If a person pushes herself very hard to go about her normal routine during these attacks, she may find *petechiae* appearing on her skin. Petechiae are tiny spots of blood which have moved to the skin surface, as if one were sweating blood. At other times blood pressure may be low (e.g., 74/52), leaving the individual fatigued and disoriented. Low body temperature is also common (e.g., 96.7).

Along with the swollen abdomen, mental symptoms that accompany hepatic porphyrias are one of the few observable signs of the condition. Anxiety and depression are both common. The individual may become disoriented, experience hallucinations or paranoia, and have no inclination to sleep. Seizures may occur in some cases.

Pain in the arms, legs, neck, and chest is common. Headaches may occur. Pain in muscles is another feature. An annoying, somewhat painful symptom is *paresthesia,* an abnormal sensation usually occurring in the arms and legs towards the hands and feet. It is somewhat similar to having one's feet or legs go to sleep, but it is a more passive feeling. It may in some cases involve numbness or lack of feeling. In other cases it may be like a tiny electrical shock that occurs in moving. The level of shock can be compared to what one receives when touching a metal object like a doorknob after walking across a carpet. The shocking paresthesias may occur in the chest and the eyes and neck when the attack is severe.

Muscle weakness is common. It may involve a specific muscle or a group. The person who has muscle weakness in one arm, for example, may find that lifting something normally lifted with ease requires more effort in that arm. Muscle weakness is one of the most serious concerns with acute intermittent porphyria because the muscle weakness may occur in the lungs, leading to respiratory failure and death.

With few exceptions an observer can see none of what is happening during these attacks. Even when all of these symptoms occur together — and they sometimes do — the sufferer can, with great effort, appear normal. When visible, the symptoms may provoke a misdiagnosis; for example, a person with mental symptoms may appear deranged. It takes a careful observer to identify correctly hepatic porphyria, either genetic or toxic.

Example of a Photosynthetic Porphyria Experience. Porphyria cutanea tarda is an example of porphyria that produces symptoms of photosensitivity. The site of the photosensitivity reaction is the skin. Sunlight produces redness and blistering on skin areas exposed to the sun, usually on the hands and face. The individual may feel pain, rather than gentle warmth, when exposed to sunshine. Blisters heal slowly, often leaving scars. Skin becomes more likely to be injured or tear when bumped or scraped. With slow healing, infection is common. Excess hair may grow on the face, and excess skin pigmentation may also occur. Skin may thicken. (See the internet at http://www.derma.med.uni-erlangen.de/bilddb/diagnose/englisch/i277140.htr for illustrations.)

It would seem that compared to acute intermittent porphyria, porphyria cutanea tarda has less severe symptoms. That is hardly the case. Mild to severe liver damage accompanies this disorder, and people with porphyria cutanea tarda may develop liver cancer.

PREVENTING PORPHYRIA ATTACKS

The key word in preventing porphyria attacks is *avoidance.* Ideally, someone with porphyria should carefully avoid anything that sets it off.

Unfortunately, there are thousands of substances that can precipitate a porphyria attack in people who have hereditary porphyria (known or latent) or induce porphyrias in otherwise healthy individuals. At least one of these substances is endogenous (produced within the body); others are exogenous (produced from sources outside the body). The endogenous substance is estrogen. Menstruation in some women can initiate a porphyria attack. In addition to estrogen, there are numbers of substances which mimic estrogen or otherwise affect the endocrine system.

Here are some examples of common household substances that can cause porphyria attacks or create porphyria in otherwise healthy individuals. Advertising has convinced us that these substances make our lives better; in truth, they can ruin the health of susceptible individuals.

ethanol	herbicides	pesticides	fungicides
alcohol (beverage)	acetone	lead	tires (butadiene)
styrene	formaldehyde	freons	hydrogen peroxide
methyl ethyl ketone	latex paint	latex glue	vinyl
plastics	dry cleaning	hair spray	petrochemicals
fluorine	perfumes	xylene	fireworks
cosmetics	cortisone	disinfectants	pharmaceuticals

There is an exhaustive list of porphyrinogenic substances maintained and for sale by Cynthia Wilson at the Chemical Injury Information Network. The address is Box 301, White Sulphur Springs, Montana 59645. For anyone who has porphyria this resource is a necessity.

Doctors need to know what substances trigger porphyria, and the lists available in the medical literature are brief. Again, the list at the Chemical Injury Information Network is a valuable resource. People with porphyria should identify themselves with identification bracelets or a card in the wallet so that in an emergency the medical condition is clear, and they should be certain that their treating physicians know what substances are porphyrinogenic. Treatment is symptomatic. Ingesting carbohydrates is helpful. Sometimes hematin or glucose is used to treat severe cases.

Finally, people with porphyria need to be prepared for doctors who, though well-meaning, may create more problems. In more than a few instances, people exhibiting neurovisceral symptoms have been given

ANTIDEPRESSANT AGENTS
Heterocyclic antidepressants

amitriptyline [1,2]	nortriptyline [1,2]	imipramine [1,2]
doxepin [5]	trimipramine [1,2]	clomipramine [1,2]
trazodone [6]	alprazolam [1]	

in the same family*: protiptyline, amoxapine, desipramine

Monoamine oxidase inhibitors

pargyline [1,2]	isocarboxazid [7]	tranylcypromine [1]

in the same family: clorgyline, phenelzine, deprenyl

ANTIANXIETY AGENTS
Benzodiazepines

meprobamate [1,2,3]	barbiturates [1,2]	hydroxyzine [1,2]
thioridazine [1,2]	alprazolam [2]	clorazepate [2]
chlordiazepoxide [1,2]	diazepam [1,2,4]	halazepam [8]
oxazepam [1,2]	prazepam [2]	

in the same family: phenothiazine

ANTIPSYCHOTIC AGENTS

chlormezanone [1,2,3]	thioridazine [1,2]

in the same family: perphenazine, haloperidol, chlorpromazine, lithium, fluphenazine, trifluoperazine, thiothixene

*Drugs in the same family should also be considered suspect. Doctors should prescribe them only with extreme caution, always remaining aware that similar drugs have been proven porphyrinogenic.

[1] M. R. Moore, et al.: *Disorders of Porphyria Metabolism,* Plenum Medical Book Company, 1987.
[2] M. R. Moore, K. E. L. McColl: "Therapy of the Acute Porphyrias," *Clinical Biochemistry,* vol. 22, June 1989.
[3] National Library of Medicine, Agency for Toxic Substances and Disease Registry: "Hazardous Substances Database — Porphyria," July 1994. (Toxnet computer search)
[4] Zakim and Boyer: *Hepatology,* 2d ed., 1990.
[5] Par Pharmaceutical, Inc.: Package insert for doxepin hydrochloride capsules, USP, Feb. 1995.
[6] S. Budavari et al., eds.: *The Merck Index: An Encyclopedia of Chemicals and Drugs,* 11th ed., 1989.
[7] R. J. Lewis, ed.: *Sax's Dangerous Properties of Industrial Materials,* 8th ed., 1994.
[8] P. L. Denniston et al., eds.: *Physicians' GenRx 1995* (Riverside, Conn.: Mosby-Year Book).

Chart 7. Psychiatric Porphyrinogenic Drugs

psychiatric drugs. These drugs as a group are highly porphyrinogenic. (See Chart 7.) The many MCS sufferers who develop asthma often experience another treatment problem: They are given steroids and inhalers which use hydrocarbon propellants (freons). Both the oral steroids and the hydrocarbon propellants are porphyrinogenic. Not only do oral steroids induce porphyria, but also they can initiate diabetes, further complicating the medical condition, since eating carbohydrates relieves porphyria symptoms.

SEPARATING INHERITED PORPHYRIAS
FROM TOXIC-INDUCED PORPHYRIAS

The question of whether a porphyria is inherited or toxic-induced usually arises in connection with issues of liability. Suppose, for example, that a person rents an apartment that becomes heavily infested by some pest. The apartment owner authorizes the apartment manager to contract out for a pest control service. The service removes the pest but also sets off a latent porphyria attack in the tenant. Now there is an economic incentive for the landlord or pest-control service to question the origin of the porphyria. A toxic-induced porphyria set off in the workplace provokes the same question. It is possible to settle this question with testing that determines whether porphyria is inherited or genetic.

Porphyria Testing. The deficit of enzymes that causes porphyria can result from either genetic factors or toxic exposure. (This is true for both acute intermittent porphyria and porphyria cutanea tarda.) Testing for porphyria can identify the excess porphyrins excreted in urine, but testing for low enzymes is necessary to determine whether the case is genetic or toxic-induced. For example, in the case depicted in Chart 6, testing for porphyrins in urine would suggest the condition was inherited porphyria cutanea tarda with symptoms of photosensitivity. If the patient in this case has blisters on the back of his hand, they might be accurately diagnosed as a symptom of his porphyria. If, however, he also has neurovisceral symptoms such as severe abdominal cramping and lethargic feelings, they might be diagnosed as a symptom of worry over his condition. That could be accurate, but it could also be a misdiagnosis stemming from the assumption that only one enzyme is deficient. While inherited porphyrias nearly always involve a single deficiency and produce only one type of symptoms, multiple enzyme deficiencies are not at all rare in toxic-induced porphyrias — and they can produce neurovisceral symptoms *in combination with* photosensitivity.

[47]

To separate inherited from acquired porphyria, then, it is necessary to test for enzyme deficiencies as well as for porphyrins in urine. Few laboratories in the United States are equipped to handle testing for multiple enzyme deficiencies. The Mayo Medical Laboratories in Rochester, Minnesota, are used nationally for solving complex porphyria cases. They have the capacity to perform multiple enzyme tests.

There is another aspect to porphyria testing. Multiple tests are important to identify whether the enzyme levels remain relatively stable, as they do in inherited porphyrias, or whether they are tied to exposure to porphyrinogenic substances, as they are in toxic-induced porphyrias. A person, who, for example, developed toxic induced porphyria at work may be able to produce a perfectly normal set of test data by staying at home for some time. The medical principle "lack of evidence is not evidence of lack" is very important here. Simply going to a grocery store could set off another attack of toxic-induced porphyria.

It is impossible to overemphasize the need for multiple enzyme testing, and testing over time, in suspected cases of toxic-induced porphyria. Porphyrins in the urine can be too easily dismissed as not indicative of a diseased state. Victims must recognize when testing is inadequate and push for the data they need.

Toxic-Induced Porphyria and Work. Once a person develops toxic-induced porphyria, he or she is at continual risk of subsequent exposures with the residual effects of active porphyria. Most of the individuals who have developed toxic-induced porphyrias at work wish they could return to work safely. Here is why they cannot:

— If the toxic-induced porphyria includes the porphyria cutanea tarda type, the person should not be exposed to sunlight, including sun through windows.

— The commute to work could set off an attack: vehicle exhaust is porphyrinogenic; states where ethanol is routinely used in gasoline add another porphyrinogenic substance.

— For those whose brains have been damaged, it is unlikely they will be able to perform at anything like their previous level. Even straining to do work well, they will probably make errors without even realizing it. Furthermore, retraining may be virtually impossible due to the parts of the brains affected (e.g., limbic structures where short term memory occurs);

— The office or industrial setting would likely set off another porphyria attack, which could be fatal; and

— Absurd though it may seem, having such a person in a workplace could be distracting, if not frightening, to other workers.

LIVING WITH PORPHYRIA: BECOMING A DECIDUOUS TREE AFTER LIFE AS AN EVERGREEN

For the MCS sufferer, a diagnosis of toxic-induced porphyria will not change the fact that he or she needs to continue coping with chemical sensitivity. The diagnosis may, however, persuade the sufferer to recognize the change in his or her "tree type." To understand what this means, it helps to realize that while people manufacture heme for the transport of oxygen in the respiratory process before expiring carbon dioxide, plants manufacture chlorophyll in the place of heme for their use of carbon dioxide before expiring oxygen in the exchange of gases. Deciduous trees require a winter resting period. Evergreens do not. Heme is to a person what chlorophyll is to a plant. Just as some plants are deciduous, some people (those with porphyria) are different from those whose heme synthesis is normal. Deciduous trees lose their leaves during winter and enter a resting phase. People with toxic-induced porphyria often discover that winter is the roughest time. Part of the reason is that instead of slowing down as deciduous trees do by shedding their leaves and entering a resting phase, people try to keep doing what they have been doing all along. In other words, they attempt to continue on as evergreens. Certainly, setting goals and objectives is worthwhile, and trying to attain them is commendable. What people with toxic-induced porphyria need to recognize is that trying to reach goals in winter may be more difficult or even impossible. Placing heavy demands on one's self in the winter can add too much stress, setting up the system for further difficulty.

HEMOPROTEINS: HEMOGLOBIN AND CYTOCHROME P-450

Heme is produced at the end of the metabolic process illustrated by Charts 3 and 4. Heme combines with other substances to produce hemoproteins such as hemoglobin and cytochromes. Their presence in appropriate number depends on the proper functioning of heme synthesis.

Hemoglobin. Hemoglobin is a protein contained in red blood cells. Hemoglobin molecules bind with oxygen, then release the oxygen into the tissues of the body. Oxyhemoglobin is the name for hemoglobin that is carrying oxygen. Oxyhemoglobin is what gives blood its red color. When oxygen is given over to cells, hemoglobin turns purplish-blue. The empty hemoglobin molecule then picks up carbon dioxide or other waste gas and takes it away for expiration from the lungs. This completes the metabolic process for exchange of gases: the carbon dioxide — oxygen cycle.

Cytochrome P-450. Cytochromes are heme-containing proteins. Cytochrome P-450 is a family of enzymes that is present in both the plant and the animal kingdom. In a single species there may be as many as 100 members of the cytochrome P-450 family. A fantastic illustration of cytochrome P-450 is available on the internet at

ftp://pdb.pdb.bnl.gov/images/GIF/8CPP_cytochrome-P450_1.gif

There are two major classes of cytochrome P-450: (1) those located in the mitochondria, which metabolize endogenous substances (for example, steroids, prostaglandins, fatty acids); and (2) those located in the smooth endoplasmic reticulum (primarily in the liver), which metabolize exogenous substances (for example, drugs, environmental pollutants, and natural plant and animal products).[44] It is in the metabolism of exogenous substances that problems relating to MCS and the porphyrias occur.

Xenobiotics and Inhibition of Cytochrome P-450. Cytochrome P-450 can be inhibited (decreased) by a variety of factors. An inherited deformity in a gene can cause a deficient state. Another means of inhibiting cytochrome P-450 is by ingesting or inhaling xenobiotics (foreign substances) that function as inhibitors. Some examples are drugs or their metabolites such as Prozac or Paxil[44] or acetaminophen.[53] Aldehydes[46] and other porphyrinogenic substances may also serve as inhibitors.[38] Inhibition of cytochrome P-450 can lead to toxic accumulations of xenobiotics. If, for example, an individual inhales or ingests a xenobiotic, whether at a low level for a long time or a high level during a brief exposure, the xenobiotic breakdown for excretion depends upon the cytochrome P-450 enzyme. Cytochrome P-450 breaks down the xenobiotic into smaller fragments which are then excreted. When cytochrome P-450 is inhibited the metabolism of the xenobiotic is slowed down. If the individual continues to ingest or inhale the substance, then the toxic accumulates because cytochrome P-450 is not able to keep up with the load. The accumulated xenobiotic then is free to wreak havoc where it will, anywhere in the body. This is not unlike the process in heme synthesis where the decreased enzyme level causes an accumulation of porphyrins.

The situation can become even worse when other xenobiotics enter the picture. Suppose a person experiencing the symptoms of toxic accumulation sees a doctor who interprets the symptoms as a depression combined with a flu. The doctor prescribes Prozac or Paxil for depression plus an antibiotic for an infection secondary to the flu. Prozac and Paxil are both porphyrinogenic and can inhibit the very enzyme activity that should clear them from the body. Many antibiotics fit the same profile. Thus these medications, taken by our hypothetical patient, increase his level of toxics significantly. Not only do the drugs themselves add to the accumulation of toxic substances, but also the delay in metabolism extends the half-life of the drugs waiting for processing. As the patient experiences continuing distress, the doctor may encourage him to continue with the drugs, assuming that the side effects will pass and not realizing that continued doses of medication are making the toxicity level serious indeed. If the toxic accumulation is porphyrinogenic, then the material may induce porphyria or, if porphyria is already present, increase the severity of the condition. Just such a scenario has been played out time and again in the MCS population.

Metabolism of Xenobiotics to Toxic Metabolites. In the normal process cytochrome P-450 breaks down exogenous substances into smaller fragments. Those fragments are reactive and may readily combine with other materials to (1) bind covalently to protein and unsaturated fatty acids or (2) induce lipid peroxidation, impairing vital cell functions such as maintaining calcium homeostasis, without which cells die or cause a hypersensitivity reaction in the liver.[30] The covalent binding of the metabolites to liver cell macromolecules creates liver lesions[43] and liver disease.[30] These metabolites may also produce indirect injury by immune-mediated membrane damage.[34]

Inhibition and Normal Metabolic Processes Combined. The creation of new forms of toxic fragments by normal metabolic processes can occur independently of a toxic accumulation caused by cytochrome P-450 inhibition, or it can occur concurrently. In some instances the metabolites themselves actually inhibit cytochrome P-450.

Cytochrome P-450 metabolizes toxins, mutagens, and carcinogens. Cytochrome P-450 can convert protoxins, promutagens, and procarcinogens to their hazardous forms. It may also clear the protoxins, promutagens, and procarcinogens from the body. Decreasing the levels of cytochrome P-450 could decrease the risk of transformation to the hazardous form, or increase the risk by decreasing the rate of clearance and permitting longer exposure to high concentrations.[44]

Induction of Cytochrome P-450. Some forms of toxic-induced porphyria can be traced to induction of cytochrome P-450.[50] (pages 96 ff) Cytochrome P-450 induction has been shown instrumental in causing porphyria when individuals have been exposed to halogenated aromatic compounds in their environment.

Chart 8 provides a summary of possible interactions between the heme biosynsthesis and cytochrome P-450 in the liver.

AN MCS MODEL

It is possible at this point to postulate a model for MCS. Chart 9 shows this model in terms of the three basic systems involved in MCS: the immune system, the central nervous system, and the endocrine system (in this case, specifically, the liver). These systems do not exist in a vacuum. They communicate with one another. Xenobiotics are ubiquitous. Humans eat them and inhale them and in some instances absorb them through skin. Inside the human body xenobiotics can have a shotgun effect on any system, organ, tissue, or cell.

The immune system. In the early years of trying to define MCS, the effects of xenobiotics were first seen in the immune system. Immune profiles showed elevated levels of interleukins, sometimes antibodies to specific xenobiotics, and autoantibodies. These data served as biomarkers of toxic exposure but failed to identify or explain the overall effect.

The central nervous system. In time the central nervous system effects became clear. Cognitive abnormalities were discovered on neuropsychological assessments, and findings of brain impairment, ranging from mild to severe, were routine. Electrochemical abnormalities could be detected on evoked potentials testing; PET scans with radioactive isotope glucose uptake showed areas where lesions prevented the brain from receiving the normal amount of glucose; SPECT scans showed abnormal blood perfusion, making it clear that the brains might be inadequately oxygenated, and in some cases vascular disease was occurring in vessels in the brain; and,

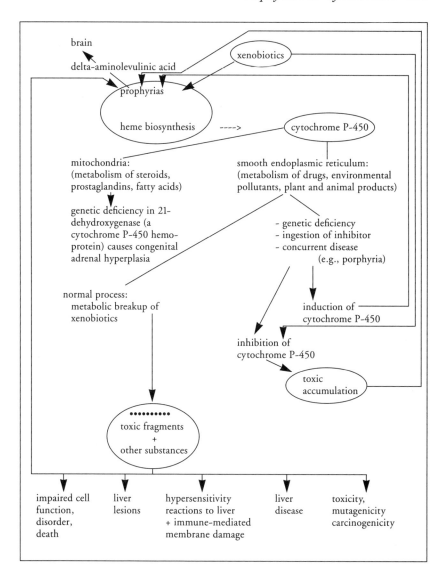

**Chart 8. Hepatic Interactions Involving Heme Biosynthesis
and Cytochrome P-450: What Can Happen**

occasionally, lesions showed up on MRIs. These data were first gathered on patients often identified as having the MCS symptom complex. Later it became apparent that military veterans returning from the Persian Gulf War were exhibiting extremely similar symptoms. The *Journal of the American Medical Association*, January 15, 1997, provides data from which the parallel in neurological symptoms can be drawn. Some Gulf War veterans have tested positive for toxic-induced porphyrias.

The liver. The resemblance between the symptom complex of MCS and that of porphyria was noticed in the mid–1990s. Testing of hundreds of people with MCS symptoms made the connection very clear. Physicians who test their MCS patient pools may find that 90 percent of the patients either test positive for toxic-induced porphyrias or have some form of porphyrinopathy. Add to that the self-perpetuating aspects of cytochrome P-450 with heme biosynthesis and the smoke begins to clear. What's more, Gulf War veterans who have been tested show striking similarities in test data with respect to porphyrias and porphyrinopathies.

The model in Chart 9 is a beginning only. It illustrates what can occur, not what must occur. With the numbers of porphyrinogenic and neurotoxic substances in the environment, this chart helps to demonstrate the self-perpetuating nature of MCS. The xenobiotics illustrated can represent more than one substance. Not all xenobiotics, for example, induce cytochrome P-450. There are some that do and some that have the reverse effect. Much that is already known could be added, and in time, even more will be known. The purpose of the model is to provide a visual depiction of how basic human processes can be set into chaos by simple encounters with day-to-day toxics. It is hoped, too, that the model will encourage others to take what they know of this symptom complex and expand the view with their own areas of expertise.

References

1. Anderson, K. E., H. L. Bradlow, S. Sassa, and A. Kappas: "Studies in porphyria. VIII. Relationship of the 5-alpha-reductive metabolism of steroid hormone to clinical expression of the genetic defect in acute intermittent porphyria." *Am J Med*, 1979; 66: 644–650.

2. Anderson, K. E., I. M. Spitz, S. Sassa, C. W. Bardin, and A. Kappas: "Prevention of cyclical attacks of acute intermittent porphyria with a long-acting agonist of luteinizing hormone–releasing hormone." *New Eng J Med*, 1984; 311: 643–645.

3. Andersson, C., and F. Lithner: "Hypertension and renal disease in patients with acute intermittent porphyria." *J Intern Med*, 1994; 236(2): 169–175.

4. Balter, P., R. C. Muehrcke, A. M. Morris, J. B. Moles, and A. G. Lawrence:

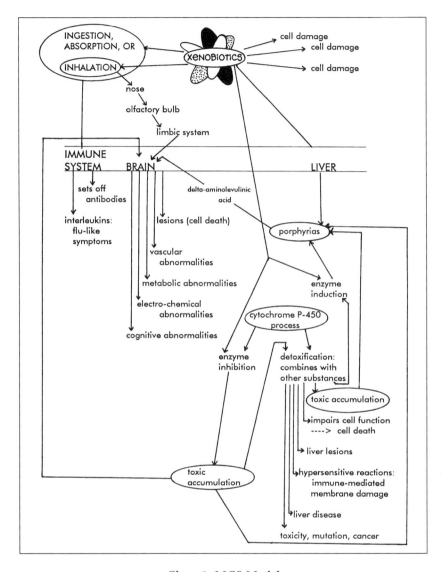

Chart 9. MCS Model

"Chronic toxic nephropathies — diagnosis and management." *Ann Clin Lab Sci*, 1976; 6(4): 306–311.

5. Beru, N., K. Sahr, and E. Goldwasser: "Inhibition of heme synthesis in bone marrow cells by succinylacetone: effect on globin synthesis." *J Cell Biochem*, 1983; 21(2): 93–105.

6. Bont, A., A. J. Steck, and U. A. Meyer: "Acute hepatic porphyria and its neurological syndrome." *Schweiz Med Wochenschr,* 1996; 126(1–2): 6–14.

7. Bottomley, S. S., H. L. Bonkowsky, and M. Kreimer-Birnbaum: "The diagnosis of acute intermittent porphyria. Usefulness and limitations of the erythrocyte uroporphyrinogen I synthase assay." *Am J Clin Pathol,* 1981; 76(2): 133–139.

8. Chalevelakis, G., C. Lyberatos, D. Manopoulos, J. Pyrovolakis, and C. Gardikas: "Erythrocyte delta-aminolaevulinic acid dehydratase, urinary porphyrins and porphyrin precursors in iron deficiency anaemia." *Acta Haematol,* 1977; 57(5): 305–309.

9. Checkoway, H., L. G. Costa, J. Camp, T. Coccini, W. E. Daniell, and R. L. Dills: "Peripheral markers of neurochemical function among styrene-exposed workers." *Br J Indus Med,* 1992; 49: 560–565.

10. Church, S. E., K. E. McColl, M. R. Moore, and G. R. Youngs: "Hypertension and renal impairment as complications of acute porphyria." *Nephrol Dial Transplant,* 1992; 7(10): 986–990.

11. Correia, M. A., D. A. Litman, and J. M. Lunetta: "Drug-induced modulations of hepatic heme metabolism. Neurological consequences." *Ann N Y Acad Sci,* 1987; 514: 248–255.

12. Costa, L. G., and L. Manzo: "Biochemical markers of neurotoxicity: research strategies and epidemiological applications." *Toxicol Lett,* 1995; 77:137–144.

13. Daya, S., K. O. Nonaka, G. R. Buzzell, and R. J. Reiter: "Heme precursor 5-aminolevulinic acid alters brain tryptophan and serotonin levels without changing pineal serotonin and melatonin concentrations." *J Neurosci Res,* 1989; 23(3): 304–309.

14. de Klerk, M., A. Weideman, C. Malan, and B. C. Shanley: "Urinary porphyrins and porphyrin precursors in normal pregnancy. Relationship to urinary total oestrogen excretion." *S Afr Med J,* 1975; 49(14): 581–583.

15. De Matteis, F., and G. S. Marks: "Cytochrome P450 and its interactions with the heme biosynthetic pathway." *Can J Physiol Pharmacol,* 1996; 74(1): 1–8.

16. Doss, M.: "Alcohol-induced changes of porphyrin metabolism." *Leber Magen Darm,* 1978; 8(5): 278–285.

17. Dumic, M.: "Congenital adrenal hyperplasia due to 21-hydroxylase enzyme deficiency." *Lijec Vjesn,* 1996: 118(S1): 13–16.

18. Echeverria, D., N. Heyer, M. D. Martin, C. A. Naleway, J. S. Woods, and A. C. Bittner: "Behavioral effects of low-level exposure to Hg among dentists." *Neurotoxicol Teratol,* 1995; 17: 161–168.

19. Ellefson, R. D., and R. E. Ford: "The Porphyrias: Characteristics and laboratory tests." *Reg Toxicol and Pharmacol,* 1996; 24: S119–S125.

20. Ezrin, C., and R. E. Kowalske: *The Endocrine Control Diet,* (New York: Harper-Collins, 1989).

21. Ferrara, R., R. Tolando, L. J. King, and M. Manno: "Cytochrome P450 inactivation during reductive metabolism of 1,1-dichloro-2,2,2-trifluoroethane (HCFC-123) by phenobarbital- and pyridine-induced rat liver microsomes." *Toxicol Appl Pharmacol,* 1997; 142(2): 420–428.

22. Frydman, R. B., E. S. Levy, A. Valasinas, and B. Frydman: "Biosynthesis of uroporphyrinogens. Interaction among 2-aminomethyltripyrranes and the enzymatic system." *Biochemistry,* 1978; 17(1): 115–120.

23. Gonzales-Ramirez, D., R. M. Maiorino, M. Zuniga-Charles, Z. Xu, K. M. Hurlburt, P. Junco-Munoz, M. M. Aposhian, R. C. Dart, J. H. Diaz Gana, D. Echeverria, and J. S. Woods: "Sodium 2,3-dimercaptopropane-1-sulfonate challenge test for mercury in humans. II. Urinary mercury, porphyrins and neurobehavioral changes of dental workers in Monterrey, Mexico." *J Pharmacol Exptl Ther,* 1995; 272: 264–274.

24. Goren, M. B., and C. Chen: "Acute intermittent porphyria with atypical neuropathy." *South Med J,* 1991; 84(5): 668–669.

25. Greenspan, G. H., and A. J. Block: "Respiratory insufficiency associated with acute intermittent porphyria." *South Med J,* 1981; 74(8): 954–956.

26. Held, H.: "Effect of alcohol on the heme and porphyrin synthesis interaction with phenobarbital and pyrazole." *Digestion,* 1977; 15(2):136–146.

27. Holloszy, J. O., and W. W. Winder: "Induction of delta-aminolevulinic acid synthase in muscle by exercise or thyroxine." *Am J Physiol,* 1979; 236(3): R180–R183.

28. Isselbacher, K. I., E. Braunwald, J. D. Wilson, J. B. Martic, A. S. Fauci, and D. L. Kasper (eds.): *Harrison's Principles of Internal Medicine,* 13th edition (New York: McGraw-Hill, 1994).

29. Juknat, A. A., M. L. Kotler, and A. M. Battle: "High delta-aminolevulinic acid uptake in rat cerebral cortex: effect on porphyrin biosynthesis." *Comp Biochem Physiol C Pharmacol Toxicol Endocrinol,* 1995; 111(1): 143–150.

30. Kaplowitz, N., T. Y. Aw, F. R. Simon, and A. Stolz: "Drug-induced hepatotoxicity." *Ann Intern Med,* 1986; 104(6): 826–839.

31. Khanderia, U., and A. Bhattacharya: "Acute intermittent porphyria: pathophysiology and treatment." *Pharmacotherapy,* 1984; 4(3): 144–150.

32. Laiwah, A. A., R. Mactier, K. E. McColl, M. R. Moore, and A. Goldberg: "Early-onset chronic renal failure as a complication of acute intermittent porphyria." *Q J Med,* 1983; 52(205): 92–98.

33. Lee, S. S., J. T. Buters, T. Pineau, P. Fernandez-Salguero, F. J. Gongalez: "Role of CYP2E1 in the hepatotoxicity of acetaminophen." *J Biol Chem,* 1996; 271(20): 12063–12067.

34. Lee, W. M.: "Review article: drug-induced hepatotoxicity." *Aliment Pharmacol Ther,* 1993; 7(5): 477–485.

35. Lin, J. L., and P. S. Lim: "Does lead play a role in the development of renal insufficiency in some patients with essential hypertension?" *J Hum Hypertens,* 1994; 8(7): 495–500.

36. Marcus, D. L., J. L. Halbrecht, A. L. Bourque, G. Lew, H. Nadel, and M. L. Freedman: "Effect of cimetidine on delta-aminolevulinic acid synthase and microsomal heme oxygenase in rat liver." *Biochem Pharmacol,* 1984; 33(13): 2005–2008.

37. Marks, G. S.: "Exposure to toxic agents: the heme biosynthetic pathway and hemoproteins as indicator." *CRC Critical Rev in Toxicol,* 1985; 15(2): 151–164.

38. McNamee, J. P., M. Jurima-Romet, S. M. Kobus, and G. S. Marks: "cDNA-expressed human cytochrome P450 isozymes. Inactivation by porphyrinogenic xenobiotics." *Drug Metab Dispos,* 1997; 25(4): 437–441.

39. Miller, D. M., and J. S. Woods: "Redox activities of mercury-thiol complexes: implications for mercury-induced porphyria and toxicity." *Chem-biol Interact,* 1993; 88:23–35.

40. Murray, M.: "Drug-mediated inactivation of cytochrome P450." *Clin Exp Pharmacol Physiol,* 1997; 24(7): 465–470.

41. Mustajoki, P., and J. Heinonen: "General anesthesia in 'inducible' porphyrias." *Anesthesiology,* 1980; 53(1): 15–20.

42. Niznikiewiez, J., and I. Jablonska-Kaszewska: "Diagnostic difficulties in acute intermittent porphyria. Report of two cases." *Pol Arch Med Wewn,* 1996, 95(6): 561–564.

43. Pessayre, D., and J. P. Benhamou: "Reactive metabolites of xenobiotics: their role in the hepatotoxicity of drugs." *C R Seances Soc Biol Fil,* 1979; 173(2): 458–468.

44. Preskorn, S. H., and R. D. Magnus: "Inhibition of hepatic P-450 isoenzymes

by serotonin selective reuptake inhibitors: In vitro and in vivo findings and their implications for patient care." *Psychopharm Bull,* 1994; 30(2): 251–259.

45. Puy, H., J. C. Deybach, P. Baudry, J. Callebert, Y. Touitou, and Y. Nordmann: "Decreased nocturnal plasma melatonin levels in patients with recurrent acute intermittent porphyria attacks." *Life Sci,* 1993; 53(8): 621–627.

46. Ranes, G. M., E. W. Chiang, A. D. Vaz, M. J. Coon: "Mechanism-based inactivation of cytochrome P4502B4 by aldehydes: relationship to aldehyde deformation via a peroxyhemiacetal intermediate." *Biochemistry,* 1997; 36(16): 4895–4902.

47. Rothman, N., M. T. Smith, R. B. Hayes, R. D. Traver, B. Hoener, S. Campleman, G. L. Li, M. Dosemeci, M. Liner, L. Zhang, L. Xi, S. Wacholder, W. Lu, K. B. Meyer, N. Titenko-Holland, J. T. Stewart, S. Yin, and D. Ross: "Benzene poisoning, a risk factor for hematological malignancy, is associated with the NQO1 609C —>T mutation and rapid fractional excretion of chlorzoxazone." *Cancer Res,* 1997; 57(14): 2839–2842.

48. Shiue, J. W., F. Y. Lee, K. J. Hsiao, Y. T. Tsai, S. D. Lee, and S. J. Wu: "Abnormal thyroid function and hypercholesterolemia in a case of acute intermittent porphyria." *Taiwan I Hsueh Hui Tsa Chih,* 1989; 88(7): 729–731.

49. Shively, B. D., J. M. Clochesy, J. P. Briones, D. L. Spositio, and J. A. Kloos: "Caring for patients with acute intermittent porphyria." *AACN Clin Issues,* 1994; 5(1): 36–41.

50. Silbergeld, E. K., and B. A. Fowler (eds.): *Mechanisms of Chemical-Induced Porphyrinopathies* (New York: The New York Academy of Sciences, 1987).

51. Shoolingin-Jordan, P. M.: "Porphobilinogen deaminase and uroporphyrinogen III synthase: structure, molecular biology, and mechanism." *J Bioenereg Biomembr,* 1995; 27(2): 181–195.

52. Siddiqui, S. M., G. S. Rao, and K. P. Pandya: "Depletion of liver regulatory heme in benzene exposed rats." *Toxicology,* 1988; 48(3): 245–251.

53. Simmonds, P. L., C. L. Luckhurst, and J. S. Woods: "Quantitative evaluation of heme biosynthetic pathway parameters as biomarkers of low level lead exposure in rats." *J Toxicol Environ Health,* 1995; 44: 351–367.

54. Snawder, J. E., A. L. Roe, R. W. Benson, and D. W. Roberts: "Loss of CYP2E1 and CYP1A2 activity as a function of acetaminophen dose: relation to toxicity." *Biochem Biophys Res Commun,* 1994; 203(1): 532–539.

55. Sugimura, K., "Acute intermittent porphyria." *Nippon Rinsho,*1995; 53(6): 1418–1421.

56. Tefferi, A., J. P. Colgan, and L. A. Solberg, Jr.: "Acute porphyrias: diagnosis and management." *Mayo Clin Proc,* 1994; 69(10): 991–995.

57. Vidt, D. G.: "Recognition and management of reversible renal failure." *South Med J,* 1994; 87(10): 1018–1027.

58. Vincent, D., J. F. Devars du Mayne, J. C. Deybach, A. Pradalier, and Y. Nordmann: "Hepatic porphyria: diagnostic and therapeutic strategies." *Rev Med Interne,* 1994; 15(8): 521–527.

59. White, P. C.: "Genetic diseases of steroid metabolism." *Vitam Horm,* 1994; 49: 131–195.

60. Wongthim, S., T. Hemachudha, and K. Punthumchinda: "Respiratory insufficiency associated with acute hepatic porphyria." *J Med Assoc Thai,* 1989; 72(11): 655–659.

II

LEGAL INFORMATION

Whether injured at work, home, school, or another place, many of the chemically injured eventually turn to attorneys for help in dealing with matters of compensation. Executive function is one of the common losses of the chemically injured, and tasks such as keeping track of critically important deadlines, complying with the demands of workers' compensation officials and Social Security administrators, and responding to legal or governmental adversaries are often beyond their ability. Attorneys can help, though all too often, the legal battles still end in defeat.

In this section, an attorney reveals how one state's legal system is weighted against the chemically injured and their claims. He goes on to suggest how the system might be restructured, and emphasizes the urgent need for change.

5. NO BALM IN GILEAD: WHY WORKERS' COMPENSATION FAILS WORKERS IN A TOXIC AGE*

Randolph I. Gordon

> *I am wounded at the sight of my people's wound;*
> *I go like a mourner, overcome with horror.*
> *Is there no balm in Gilead, no physician there?*
>
> Jeremiah 8:21–22

THE STORY

For over a decade, my office had a nook: a leather loveseat with a shelf and bookcase behind it, an oval wood coffee table, and two tall wingback chairs. Its form matched its function nearly perfectly. Intended to provide a safe place for my clients to unburden themselves, it saw a steady stream of women and men doing just that. Many a day I waved a husband and wife towards the loveseat. Without prompting, the wife would describe a pattern of symptoms with which I would come to be all too familiar: crushing headaches, eye irritation, nosebleeds, sore throat, painful and difficult breathing, fatigue, thirst, nausea, increased emotionality, insomnia, impaired

*Note: A version of this article was published in March 1996 by the *Washington State* Bar News, *whom the author wishes to thank for their support. The author must also acknowledge with thanks the insights offered by James D. Hailey and his inestimable contribution as co-counsel representing plaintiffs in *Birklid v. Boeing.

memory, inability to cope, loss of interest in things usually enjoyed, decreased sexual interest, trouble concentrating, and sensitivity to certain materials.

The symptoms first arose when the client was exposed to certain materials in the workplace. When she worked a long week her symptoms would worsen; after a three-day weekend her symptoms would improve. It took awhile for her to associate her symptoms with the workplace because she had been working overtime consistently for months — and because the company denied knowledge of any ill effects from exposure. Medical records confirmed her having reported these symptoms on numerous occasions. Her fellow workers, mostly women, also felt sick. Everybody assumed it was a flu bug going around. But for some, the symptoms persisted — and worsened. For these workers, symptoms reappeared whenever they were exposed to certain substances present in the everyday environment of modern society: aftershave, gasoline, detergent, toner from photocopiers. For these workers, the path through each day had become a maze in which certain commonplace exposures had to be avoided.

As the wife would start talking about increased emotionality, I would glance over to the husband and receive the expected confirmation. He would look towards his wife with his eyes filling with tears. She needs this job, she would say. Then he would lower his eyes again.

The nook is no longer there. Yet the stream of injured visitors continues.

These people are telling a story, variations of which I have now heard countless times from factory workers, office workers, doctors, teachers, painters, and chemists. Over the years, dozens of working men and women, fearful of losing their jobs, have sat before me telling the story. The insidious onset of the constellation of symptoms. Trooping from doctor to doctor, specialist to specialist, with no explanation, no cure.

• A young man just a month or so before his wedding is unable to work. His fiancee breaks off the engagement because, as he puts it, he doesn't appear to have much of a future anymore.

• A chemist just out of school cannot look forward to the job for which he has trained for years. He learns from co-workers that the woman who sat at his desk just before him also can no longer work. She also told the story. We thought that's just the way she was, you know, having lots of problems, they tell him. But now you. His co-workers are worried.

- A top-flight, high-powered executive can no longer perform his sales job for a television network.

- A physician who once could remember the blood pressures of a full schedule of patients when writing up his office notes now has trouble remembering where he is going between examination rooms.

They all tell their own versions of the story.

I have not been trained to answer their questions. And, theoretically, as a lawyer, I do not have to. But, as a human being, I must try.

INSIDE THE BELTWAY

On March 6, 1989, at 10:00 A.M., Senator Reid of Nevada, chair of the United States Senate Subcommittee on Toxic Substances, Environmental Oversight, Research and Development, called to order the first hearing on "Worker Exposure to Toxic Materials in the Aerospace Industry."[1] In his opening remarks, the senator stated:

> I intend to set a standard for these hearings. The work place should not be a test tube and the company employees should not be guinea pigs. We cannot tolerate stone-age protections for space-age dangers. At the same time, we must do everything possible to maintain the current high standards of national security that come from extraordinary leaps forward in scientific research and available technology.
>
> Today we begin a dialogue that includes testimony from affected workers, medical experts, representatives of the aerospace industry, union officials and federal regulators. I sincerely appreciate their willingness to appear before our panel and look forward to hearing their remarks.
>
> In World War Two, we glorified Rosie the Riveter. Thirty years later, we buried her because nobody had known about the dangers of asbestos contamination. The employees of the aerospace industry protect us by the work they perform. We owe them the very same high level of protection.[2]

The sentiments expressed by the senator articulate what most Americans would regard as the expected — and appropriate — policy respecting workplace safety: Human beings ought not to be exposed to chemicals whose effects are unknown. Such a policy is beguiling in its humanity and simplicity. But is it the policy of the United States government?

It is to the dedication of the bureaucrat functioning within the constraints of his agency that we may fairly attribute most of the success of regulatory efforts, however well-conceived the underlying legislation. The testimony before the Senate subcommittee from Leo Carey, director of the Office of Field Programs of the Occupational Safety and Health Administration (OSHA),[3] and Charles Elkins, director of the Office of Toxic Substances of the Environmental Protection Agency (EPA), exemplifies both the dedication and the necessarily circumscribed perspective of the civil servant.

Consider briefly the testimony of Mr. Carey:

> [A]s a young boy I experienced the effects of occupational injuries and illnesses. I come from a small town in the anthracite region of Pennsylvania. I have had relatives killed in the mines, and I have had relatives develop black lung. I have spent the 20 years of my professional life devoted to protecting workers from injuries and illnesses.
>
> OSHA has responsibility for approximately 80 million workers in nearly 6 million work places. We are largely a field organization with an annual budget of approximately $250 million a total staff of 2400, more than 80 percent of whom are located in ten regional and 86 area and district offices throughout the country.
>
> Our mission is to assure, so far as possible, safe and healthful working conditions for every working man and woman in the nation....
>
> In the past fiscal year, federal OSHA and the states, together, have inspected approximately two and a half percent of the six million workplaces covered by OSHA.[4]

As one might expect from the administrators of government agencies, the testimony had two basic thrusts: the efficiency of the agency given existing funding levels and the inadequacy of the present level of appropriations. One would hardly expect OSHA or EPA officials to testify that it is impossible to protect the worker. We can rely upon the proffered data, but any judgment regarding the efficacy of an agency's efforts or the possibility of its attaining its expressed goals is the responsibility of an informed citizenry.

The notion that the workplace ought not to be a "test tube" for experimentation on human "guinea pigs" is so widely held that we are in danger of persuading ourselves that reality conforms with our expectations. It does not.

TOO FEW WHITE MICE

Ironically, to this observer, the testimony from the OSHA and EPA representatives did not establish justification for additional funding so much as demonstrate the futility of attempting to gain adequate knowledge through testing.

Responsibility for the policing of the Hazard Communication Standard rests with OSHA[5] and its associated agencies at the state level. The standard, first effective in May 1986, requires chemical manufacturers and importers to evaluate the hazards of the chemicals they produce or import. They must then inform their employees, as well as the employers to whom they ship their products, of the hazards. This communication, in the form of a material safety data sheet (MSDS), identifies the product, the risks associated with its use, and the appropriate protective measures. The data sheets must be available to the employees on their shifts.

The employer is required to train employees to understand the information the standard makes available to them. Training is to be provided at the time of an employee's initial assignment and whenever a new hazard is introduced into the work area. Such training must address how to read and interpret information on labels and material safety data sheets and how to detect the presence of hazardous chemicals.

Presently, the standard covers more than 575,000 chemical substances and products. OSHA has established permissible exposure limits for only 600 industrial chemicals and substances. In a written submission to the Senate subcommittee, Mr. Carey stated: "In a recent landmark effort, the agency set limits for 164 substances that had not previously been regulated by OSHA, and adopted more protective limits for 212 chemicals."[6] In the event no specific limits exist, the General Duty Clause of the Occupational Safety and Health Act (Section 5 [a] [1]) authorizes OSHA to issue citations where the employer has failed to furnish employment or place of employment free from recognized health hazards. A penalty of up to $1,000 may be proposed and up to $10,000 for each instance of a willful or repeated violation.

At present, the introduction of new chemicals in the workplace has outstripped all efforts to establish permissible exposure limits. Under the Toxic Substances Control Act (TSCA),[7] manufacturers intending to manufacture or import a new chemical are required to give 90-day advance notification to the EPA. This Premanufacture Notification (PMN) is intended to permit the EPA to evaluate the new chemical. Section 5 of TSCA requires the submission of toxicity test data that are available, but does not require toxicity testing by the manufacturer. More than 11,600 PMN submissions were received through the end of fiscal year 1988; more than half lacked any test data; fewer than 15 percent of the notices contain information respecting any effects beyond acute lethality or local irritation.[8] The PMN submissions add to the backlog of over 65,000 chemicals already in use for which health risk assessments have yet to be made. As Mr. Elkins noted:

> [T]he *Existing* Chemical Program deals with chemicals that have well-established and often major roles in the economy. To responsibly place significant restrictions on the use or manufacture of chemicals basic to the operation of the American economy requires EPA to perform extensive analyses of options and impacts....
>
> In order to regulate existing chemicals, TSCA requires EPA to make a determination that the manufacture, distribution, processing, use or disposal *will* present an unreasonable risk to health or the environment....[9]
>
> With existing chemicals, we have a much bigger problem. There are almost 65,000 chemicals in commerce. Many of these have production volumes over a billion pounds, and for many others, millions of people are exposed.[10]

It is evident that, of necessity, the efficacy of regulatory efforts rests almost entirely upon the voluntary cooperation of industry and employers. The most rigorous imaginable enforcement falls far short of that required to insure compliance in millions of workplaces for thousands of chemicals lacking any permissible exposure guidelines. Moreover, enforcement of permissible exposure limits may well require technology not yet available.

Even if we could assume vigorous enforcement and enthusiastic compliance with all the applicable regulations, the problems facing protection of workers from toxic chemical exposures in the workplace would dwarf our current scientific and medical knowledge. Even where established, permissible exposure limits generally govern individual chemicals and may not adequately protect workers in workplace situations if chemicals are introduced in the form of composites where identification of the chemical constituents and by-products may be impossible. Based upon the number of chemicals alone, analysis of the additive and synergistic effects of all combinations of these chemicals would involve more white mice than exist on earth.

As recently noted by a University of Washington investigator of one case involving phenol formaldehyde resins:

> The results of the various investigations were not surprising, particularly in view of the fact that there are no universally agreed upon methods for determining standards for exposures to mixtures containing more than a few individual compounds. In addition, some of the atmospheric collection and analytical techniques utilized to assess potential exposures are not always entirely effective. This is especially true for complex mixtures involving resin, some formulations of which were developed for use in the production of composites.
>
> A number of technical difficulties are apparent. In many instances, some resin by-products may not be collected; others, if collected, cannot be identified. Furthermore, the toxicity data for some of the identified components may be sparse or absent.[11]

Phenol formaldehyde resins are used in some common wood composites such as plywood and particle board, and phenolic-bonded laminates are used industrially and for home and office decorations. Phenolic resins are present in products such as brake linings and clutch facings and are used in paints, varnishes, rubber cement, nail lacquer and hardener, watch bands, fabrics, shoes, and, in the form of phenolic foam, flower arranging.[12] Although one might hope that the chemical constituents of such resins would be well understood given their use in factories, offices, cars, homes, cosmetics, and apparel, such is not the case. In fact, as recently as 1985, eleven new skin sensitizers were identified in such resins.[13]

MISAPPLICATION OF SCIENCE: "WHEN I HEARD THE LEARN'D ASTRONOMER"

In his poem "When I Heard the Learn'd Astronomer," Walt Whitman tells how

> When the proofs, the figures, were ranged in columns before me,
> When I was shown the charts and diagrams, to add, divide, and measure them,
> When I sitting heard the astronomer where he lectured with much applause in the lecture-room,
> How soon unaccountable I became tired and sick,

> Till rising and gliding out I wander'd off by myself,
> In the mystical moist night-air, and from time to time,
> Look'd up in perfect silence at the stars.

So, too, we often see how statistics such as permissible exposure levels and threshold limit values squeeze all the life out of the questions they seek to answer. In the final analysis, looking at the data, we are forced to ask: Of what value is it? What do PELs and TLVs tell us about an individual's susceptibility to toxic insult? The answer: not much.

Those defending employers against claims of injured workers often ignore the underlying human issues. This, perhaps, may be expected of those in service to the corporate defendants. But such defenses are based upon a misapplication of basic concepts respecting PELs and threshold limit values (TLVs). The defense, for instance, routinely will assert that a given individual could not have been injured because the exposure level was below the PEL. To understand the fallacy of this assertion requires us to understand what such figures really mean.

TLVs, established by the TLV Committee of the American Conference of Governmental Industrial Hygienists (ACGIH), were intended as unofficial guidelines for acceptable exposure. Yet they have been widely applied as official limits, and nearly 90 percent of the PELs are based directly upon the TLVs.

The TLVs are subject to change. "Each year some of the values are changed, and in a majority of instances they are reduced, sometimes to one-half or one-tenth of their previous value.... TLVs for such chemicals as benzene, vinyl chloride, and methyl chloride [have] come down from early values of 100 ppm, 500 ppm and 20,000 ppm [Cook 1945] to current levels of 10 ppm, 5 ppm and 1000 ppm," wrote S. A. Roach and S. M. Rappaport in the *American Journal of Industrial Medicine*.[14] The authors conclude that TLVs reflect the levels of exposure which were perceived at the time to be achievable in industry.

The defense consistently assumes that if exposures fall beneath certain established levels, then injury cannot occur. The ACGIH, however, has never contended that the TLVs protect all workers, even giving them the greatest conceivable weight. In fact, annually, the following language is included in the ACGIH documentation of threshold limit values:

> Because of a wide variation in individual susceptibility ... a small percentage of workers may experience discomfort from some substances at

concentrations at or below the threshold limit: a smaller percentage may be affected more seriously by aggravation of a pre-existing condition or by development of an occupational illness.[15]

According to one recent study, the incidence of adverse effects *at* the threshold limit value ranged from zero to 100 percent.[16] In other words, some TLVs are levels at which 100 percent of those exposed are adversely affected. Overall, it appears that about 14 percent of workers experience adverse effects at or below the TLV.[17] Clearly, test measurements of levels below the PELs do not negate the possibility of injury or illness.

From a scientific standpoint, *even if*: (1) all the sources of contamination were identified; (2) all the toxic chemicals were identified; (3) all such chemicals were tested under circumstances precisely replicating the environment in which the exposure occurred; and (4) all levels detected by such testing were below the TLVs and PELs, the causal relationship between exposure and injury could not be negated by the logic employed by the defense. The fact that these assumptions are not correct makes the argument put forward by the defense unscientific and invalid.

The Roach and Rappaport critical analysis of TLVs concludes:

> Since so many TLVs for chemical substances appear to offer relatively little protection, we recommend that occupational hygienists and other health professionals routinely investigate the *Documentation* and, more importantly, the reference materials pertaining to particular contaminants rather than accepting on faith that every TLV provides the protection claimed by the ACGIH.[18]

The process for setting TLVs has also been criticized.[19] Although the TLV Committee, which consists of volunteers operating on a limited budget, deserves respect for its efforts to set TLVs where none had existed, it must be pointed out that initially there was little or no experimental evidence, so the levels were based on those obtainable by industry. Castleman and Ziem cite significant or complete reliance upon unpublished corporate correspondence in a substantial proportion of cases and note that corporate representatives served as consultants to the committee. They properly caution against undue corporate influence on values which are, after all, being imposed upon the corporations themselves. The authors note, "It has … been widely recognized that the TLVs for chemical substances are in most cases poorly supported by scientific evidence."[20] They conclude that "the numerical values for exposure limits selected as 'acceptable'" are determined by "very much a political as well as a scientific process."[21]

The epidemiological data supporting the TLVs are not based on double-blind, peer-reviewed human studies. Anecdotal evidence, studies involving small numbers of individuals, animal studies, unpublished corporate correspondence, and industrial practicality all figure in establishing the limits. It is not surprising that injured workers cannot often establish injury through double-blind epidemiological studies when the TLVs and PELs upon which the defense rests its claims are themselves seldom supported in that way. When epidemiological data are available, they nearly always arise from the exposures experienced by white male, blue-collar workers in manufacturing facilities. Such data must be looked at with some care before they can be applied to other workers. Ethical and economic factors also hamper the generation of epidemiologic studies on humans.

Perhaps most significantly, there is no scientific basis for applying the TLVs and PELs to *mixtures* of chemicals. TLVs and PELs are established for single chemical exposures. They do not take into account the additive or synergistic effects of chemicals or chemical mixtures. For instance, levels of toluene at 60 percent TLV added to levels of xylene at 60 percent TLV would have an additive effect, yet the mixture would still be below the TLV for each chemical individually. The application of single chemical TLVs and PELs to circumstances of probable multiple chemical exposures is in most cases not scientifically sound. From the standpoint of the scientific method, exposures to individual contaminants below the TLVs would not in any way rule out the potential for adverse health effects to be causally related to the environment.

CONSIDERING SCIENTIFIC CAUSATION

Participants in the regulatory and compensatory framework attempting to establish the cause of toxic injuries find themselves caught in a conflict between good law and good science. Existing compensatory schemes in the State of Washington, for example, require that the injured worker establish that the injury was proximately caused by the toxic exposure in the workplace — and do so within the applicable statute of limitations governing occupational disease.[22] One commentator has pointed out that a statute of limitations on toxic substance litigation runs counter to the policies behind tort law: Time bars on ordinary torts promote efficient and accurate factual determinations, but toxic tort claims force claimants to seek compensation in the absence of the best scientific evidence and before the nature and extent of injury has been established.[23]

In cases where employees are exposed to novel mixtures of chemicals, the best scientific evidence is almost never available when needed. This is hardly surprising in light of the more than 4,000,000 mixtures, formulations, and blends estimated to have been registered with the EPA under the TSCA.[24] Moreover, even without undue pessimism, it is improbable that such scientific knowledge is ever likely to become available when needed, so long as toxicological and epidemiological studies must rely upon animal and human studies, due to the latency periods involved in exposures to subacute levels of chemicals.[25]

Epidemiology deals with the study of diseases within a subject population and may permit investigators to reach conclusions respecting the effects of actual chemical exposure upon groups of individuals. Such studies may eliminate the necessity of analogizing from animal studies or from similar chemicals, but involve creating analogies between more or less comparable human populations which leave such studies open to attack.[26] Obviously, a truly novel chemical formulation cannot have been the subject of epidemiological studies to help establish causation in a particular case. Assuming, however, that some analogy may be drawn to the effects of some of the known chemical constituents of the formulation or a similar mixture, such studies may be of only limited value to the injured worker.

> Even when epidemiological studies are able to determine very accurately excess risks of disease in populations, they are not able to determine which individuals in those populations would not have developed the disease without occupational exposure. In many cases, this uncertainty cannot be resolved.[27]

Moreover, not infrequently, epidemiological studies are unable to meet the high scientific burden required to establish a statistical association and fail to show any increased risk. In such cases,

> [c]ourts may erroneously assume, for example, that a showing of no increased risk eliminates any possibility of causation. In fact, such a showing may be related to difficulties inherent in epidemiology rather than the absence of a causal link.[28]

[71]

In *Ferebee v. Chevron Chemical Company*, the court stated that "a cause and effect relationship need not be clearly established by animal or epidemiology studies before a doctor can testify that in his opinion such a relationship exists."[29] From an evidentiary standpoint, in the absence of toxicological or epidemiological data, the ability of the injured worker to demonstrate the existence of an occupational disease rests almost entirely upon the ability of the treating physician to identify the constellation of symptoms the worker reports as the clinical manifestations of exposure to novel chemical formulations at levels able to be established.[30] Thus it can be most difficult, for both physician and patient, if novel chemicals give rise to new clinical entities which have not yet been widely recognized by the medical establishment.

The worker does not have only to be concerned with the conservatism of the medical establishment. Judicial opinions have questioned whether a treating physician can provide accurate testimony respecting causation without reliance upon epidemiological studies.[31] Such opinions seem to indicate that the injured worker must escape an impossible circularity to meet the burden of proof: In the absence of epidemiological and scientific studies, the worker must rely upon the testimony of his or her doctor; yet, the testimony of the doctor will not be permitted in the absence of supporting epidemiological and scientific studies. As a number of commentators have noted, such a conclusion would, in effect, raise the injured worker's burden of proof above the legal standard of "preponderance of the evidence" or "more likely than not" to one of "scientific certainty."[32]

The injured individual must labor under not only the honest burden of proof assumed by a plaintiff in civil litigation, but an enhanced burden imposed upon him or her by a defense none too scrupulous about the application of scientific principle. For instance, the defense may insist upon a scientific standard of proof that no one could sustain, such as requiring that a dose-response relationship be applied to a novel toxic mixture for which the dose may be impossible to establish. Toxicological principles of dose-response and specificity cannot be applied to complex mixtures, and the "science" of any defense insisting upon such application is unsound. A common example of a complex mixture is diesel exhaust. According to NIOSH: "Estimates indicate that as many as 18,000 different substances from the combustion process can be adsorbed onto diesel exhaust particulates."[33] Testing cannot come close to measuring such exposures to plaintiffs: "Exposure to diesel exhaust is difficult to measure because of the complex nature of the exhaust."[34] The same principle holds true for any complex mixture.

If defense experts nonetheless insist that a dose-response relationship and specificity of response to each chemical be established, it is worth noting that it has been held that these matters raise questions of fact best left to the jury:

> The dose-response relationship at low levels of exposure for admittedly toxic chemicals ... is one of the most sharply contested questions currently being debated in the medical community, see generally Leape, Quantitative Risk Assessment in Regulation of Environmental Carcinogens, 4 *HARVARD ENVT'L L. REV.* 86, 100–103 (1980); *surely it would be rash for a court to declare as a matter of law that, below a certain threshold level of exposure, dermal absorption of paraquat has no detrimental effect. We therefore conclude that there was sufficient evidence of causation to justify submission of that issue to the jury.* [Emphasis added.][35]

In addressing exposures to diesel exhaust and other mixtures, one must consider a veritable "chemical soup" in which the worker has been submerged. The exposed individual experiences ingestion and respiration of the offending substance; dermal contact; and direct irritation to eyes, mucous membranes, and skin from particulates. The effects of such exposures include, among others, offensive odors, chemical effects, and the mechanical, irritating effects associated with particulate matter.

The physical state of the constituents may include gaseous fumes, particulates, and the chemicals adsorbed onto particulates and respired deeply into the lungs. The potential exposures to a single chemical vary widely depending upon the routes of exposure, toxicity, and states of the chemical (gas, liquid, particulate, solution, aerosol mist). This makes calculation of precise dosage difficult even for a single chemical. Precise calculation of dosage of a complex chemical mixture is likely to be impossible. Furthermore, dose-response relationships are not applicable to chemical mixtures because of the additive or synergistic (or even offsetting) effects. Finally, specificity of response by the patient to a specific chemical cannot be determined when the patient has been exposed to a complex chemical mixture. For all these reasons, principles of dose-response and specificity are not applicable to a situation where the worker was exposed to a complex chemical mixture. Such principles are also inapplicable where the precise route, duration, and extent of toxic exposures are unable to be determined, oftentimes due to the limitations of the air tests conducted at the time.

[73]

Ironically, the "science" propounded by those defending against claims of chemical injury is often based upon professional skepticism disguised as science. Defense experts, having no burden to establish causation, need only be doubting Thomases. This role may be revealed by their inability to address or explain the evidence. Most seem able only to attack the "provability" of the injured worker's case.

The methods for establishing the causal link between novel exposures and novel diseases may involve expert witnesses expressing opinions which run contrary to those of the scientific or medical establishment. Often, the opinions of the "establishment" under scrutiny are no sounder for having been generally accepted than the proposition put forth on behalf of the injured plaintiff.

DAUBERT AND JUNK SCIENCE: COPERNICUS UNMUZZLED

The recent United States Supreme Court decision in *Daubert v. Merrell Dow Pharmaceuticals, Inc.*[36] appears to discard the *Frye* standard requiring that evidence or testimony, in order to be admissible, have "general acceptance" in the scientific community. Instead, the Court chose to admit evidence based upon an ER 702[37] inquiry into a number of factors: (1) Is the theory testable, and has it been tested? (2) Has the theory been subjected to peer review and publication? (3) What is the known or potential error rate associated with the scientific technique employed? (4) Is the technique or methodology well-known, and has it met with widespread acceptance?

This case authority suggests that the Court is moving toward acceptance of expert testimony based upon sound, but not necessarily generally *accepted*, scientific principles. If so, the door may be opening to a more liberal admission of scientific evidence. In other words, sound scientific method may be heard as testimony, even if it yields an unpopular conclusion: Copernicus *can* testify that the earth orbits around the sun, despite the weight of established opinion to the contrary.

The Washington Court of Appeals (Division I) in *Intalco Aluminum v. Dep't. of Labor and Industries*,[38] citing *Ferebee*, held that "expert testimony [must] be based on methods accepted in the scientific community" but that "an expert physician's opinion on causation need not be generally accepted in the scientific community." In *Intalco*, the court found the extensive neurologic testing by plaintiffs' physicians to be immune from attack.

In *Ferebee*,[39] the court approved of the "basic methodology," which employed tissue samples, standard tests, and patient examinations. In *Bruns v. PACCAR, Inc.*,[40] the court approved of reliance on experts for air sampling, chemical analysis, clinical examinations, and questionnaires. (See the following section, "Products Liability Actions," for further discussion of *Bruns*.)

There would seem, then, to be little disagreement that taking a detailed patient history, conducting physical examinations, having blood samples drawn and reviewed by reliable laboratories, reviewing air test results, considering the significance of a "cluster" of similar exposures and reports of illness, and exploring the medical and scientific literature constitute sound methodology. Often, the debate by those denying chemical injury appears limited to "We disagree with your conclusions."

In *Intalco*, the Washington Court of Appeals wrote: "We agree with the *Ferebee* court that the requirement that expert medical testimony be based on methods generally accepted in the scientific community pertains to the *methods* used by, not the conclusions of, the expert witness."[41] Even in pre–*Daubert* cases, it was clear that the conclusions of the experts were reserved for the jury to consider on their merits.

Causation in novel chemical injury claims can seldom be established with *scientific* certainty. In the absence of toxicological or epidemiological data, the injured worker must rely upon the evaluation of his treating physician. "In workers' compensation cases, the court must give special consideration to the opinion of the attending physician."[42] The attending physician is seldom in a position to identify occupational diseases arising from novel chemical compounds based on an isolated presentation by his or her patient. Only rarely will the attending physician have information respecting a number of workers from a common site manifesting a similar constellation of symptoms. This information is uniquely available to the in-house physician of the employer in the case of larger employers. Unfortunately, the employer's medical staff are all too rarely supportive of the workers.

The attending physician, however, will generally be safe in expressing opinions based upon *clinical* diagnoses consistent with the symptoms associated with a toxic exposure. The problem, once more, is determining which symptoms are associated with exposure to novel chemical combinations. The analysis at this point generally devolves to a debate respecting permissible exposure limits, test levels, and the completeness of the material safety data sheet provided by the manufacturer respecting the products or chemicals at issue. *Intalco* again proves exceedingly helpful respecting both the impact of chemical combinations and permissible exposure limits. The *Intalco* court concluded that the injured worker is not required to prove that a precise chemical caused the injury, so long as the evidence establishes that the conditions of the workplace were the major contributing cause of the disability.[43] The court also concluded that PELs respecting safe levels for the average worker were of no matter; the concern was the effects of exposure on the particular affected worker.[44]

PRODUCT LIABILITY ACTIONS: PROXIMATE CAUSE REVISITED

The defense will often seek to have a chemical injury case treated as though it involved a pharmaceutical product. Cases involving pharmaceuticals must consider whether the product causes injury if administered at the therapeutic dosage prescribed by a physician.[45] This question is entirely inappropriate for chemical injury cases. There is no therapeutic dosage for formaldehyde, toluene diisocyanate, diesel fuel, or other fumes or mixtures. Furthermore, in cases involving pharmaceuticals, in contrast to the toxic chemical exposures in homes, schools, and workplaces, there is no opportunity for lay (non-expert) testimony; there are no eye witnesses to the biochemistry of the drug at work.

Under the doctrine of *Erie R.R. v. Tompkins*,[46] substantive state law of products liability is properly applied with respect to chemicals in defective products. In the recent Washington case of *Bruns v. PACCAR,* a design defect products liability action, the Washington Court of Appeals addressed a case involving a "chemical soup" affecting drivers of new trucks.

In *Bruns*, 13 truck drivers who transported trucks manufactured by defendant Kenworth reported health problems which arose during and after driving the new trucks. Their symptoms included skin rashes, respiratory problems, nosebleeds, tight chests, numb fingers, headaches, and fatigue. The drivers maintained that multiple airborne chemicals in the trucks made them ill. Several air quality consultants investigated the situation but were

[76]

unable to pinpoint a specific chemical agent as the cause of the harm. One physician conducted clinical examinations and reviewed records and concluded that the symptoms were caused by an unspecified irritant "while driving newly-manufactured Kenworth trucks on a more probable than not basis."[47] She concluded that low levels or combinations of chemicals could have an irritant effect. A second physician likewise noted a more-probable-than-not association between the symptoms and work activities and "reported that some of the symptoms appeared consistent with irritation by some unidentified airborne chemical substance."[48] A NIOSH investigator, Dr. McCammon, "identified over 100 organic compounds in small quantities and found hydrocarbon, carbon monoxide, aldehydes, fiberglass, isocynates, and xylene in concentrations at less than 10 percent of their TLV and PEL."[49] "Dr. McCammon concluded: 'No single contaminant or set of conditions was identified to explain the truck drivers' health complaints.' [H]e found the temporal patterns reported by drivers consistent with a work-related etiology."[50]

Defendant PACCAR moved for summary judgment based on the drivers' failure (1) to identify chemicals in the trucks approaching threshold limit values (TLV), and (2) to establish a more-probable-than-not causal link. The trial court granted summary judgment. The Court of Appeals reversed:

> [T]he elements of a design defects products liability claim are (1) a manufacturer's product (2) that was not reasonably safe as designed (3) caused harm to the plaintiff. RCW 7.72.030(1). To establish a prima facie case under the statute, plaintiff must offer admissible evidence showing each of the elements.
> [T]o establish a design defect products liability claim a plaintiff must show that the product was not reasonably safe as designed. RCW 7.72.030(1)(a). A plaintiff may demonstrate this by ... show[ing] that, at the time of manufacture, the likelihood and seriousness of harm caused by the product outweighed the manufacturer's cost and opportunity to design a product that would not have caused the harm.... Alternatively, the plaintiff may establish manufacturer liability by showing the product was unsafe as contemplated by a reasonable consumer.
> ...The parties agree that no specific chemical emerged as the source of injury and that chemicals present in the truck cabs registered in quantities much lower than required by regulations. PACCAR contends that this would cause the jury to engage in pure speculation when undertaking the consumer expectation or risk-utility analysis.
> The drivers argue that *neither the risk-utility nor the consumer expectation*

test requires proof of a specific chemical as the design defect. We agree. A plaintiff need not prove defectiveness separately from unreasonable dangerousness.[51] [Emphasis added.]

Here, the drivers point to a "chemical soup" as the defect. They provide a list of chemicals found in the truck cabs and the concentrations at which they were found. *Therefore, we find that the drivers offered sufficient evidence to allow a reasonable person to find the trucks not reasonably safe.*[52] [Emphasis added.]

The Court of Appeals found the expert opinions correlating the exposure to the new Kenworth trucks to the drivers' injuries sufficient to avoid a jury having to engage in speculation to find proximate cause.[53]

A LAST LOOK AT CAUSATION: WHERE COMMON SENSE MEETS SCIENTIFIC SKEPTICISM

There is a wealth of evidence respecting causation which relies upon such time-tested sources of evidence as human observation, experience, sight, smell, taste, touch, and common sense.[54] The defense in a chemical injury case usually seeks to move the issue of causation to a purely "scientific" realm where such common sense lay evidence is subordinated to inappropriate toxicological and epidemiological studies where the skepticism of the defense finds support — or, at least, where an attempt can be made to increase the plaintiff's burden from a preponderance of the evidence to a scientific certainty.

In *Intalco Aluminum v. Labor & Industries,* the Washington Court of Appeals held that "the plaintiff should not be denied recovery simply because the precise etiological link between the plaintiff's disease and a specific toxin or toxins in the workplace has not yet been made."[55] The Court of Appeals specifically noted that "the absence of studies linking [plaintiff's exposure] to neurologic disease does not compel the conclusion that the claimants failed to make a showing of proximate cause."[56]

Both *Bruns* and *Italco* cite with approval the following language from *Earl v. Cryovac,*[57] in which the Idaho Court of Appeals rejects the defense argument that the failure by plaintiff's experts to specify which of the chemical components of the plastic vapor caused the injury to the plaintiff defeats the plaintiff's claims:

We do not consider it fatal to the plaintiff's case that the etiology of his disease has not been traced to a discrete component or set of components with the heated plastic vapor. As explained by our Supreme Court in *Farmer v. International Harvester Co.* [97 Idaho 742, 553 P.2d 1306 (1976)], the plaintiff need only show that the product is unsafe; he need not identify and prove the specific defects which render it unsafe. The same approach is reflected in the cases ... where victims of "meatwrapper's asthma" have been allowed to recover despite scientific uncertainty as to the precise etiological link between their disease and specific chemical(s) in the heated plastic vapors.

Even the cases often cited by the defense do not contend that toxicological evidence is required to establish scientific causation. *Daubert II,*[58] the remand of *Daubert I* to the Ninth Circuit Court of Appeals by the United States Supreme Court, involved proof that a drug (Bendectin) caused birth defects was necessarily based on a statistical analysis. Even there, however, the kind of evidence often available to those in workplace or school environments who have sustained toxic injury would be persuasive:

Not knowing the mechanism whereby a particular agent causes a particular effect is not always fatal to a plaintiff's claim. Causation can be proved even when we don't know precisely how the damage occurred, if there is sufficiently compelling proof that the agent must have caused the damage somehow.... If 50 people who eat at a restaurant one evening come down with food poisoning during the night, we can infer that the restaurant's food probably contained something unwholesome, even if none of the dishes is available for analysis. This inference is based on the fact that, in our health-conscious society, it is highly unlikely that the 50 people who have nothing in common except that they ate at the same restaurant would get food poisoning from independent sources.[59]

The existence of a common pattern of illness among affected schoolchildren or workers (or even family members), all linked closely and repeatedly with a toxic exposure, can sometimes provide precisely such compelling proof. Continuing the analogy to food poisoning, the defense is contending that testing the *reverse* side of the plate revealed nothing.[60]

Each case must be considered on its unique set of facts. Consider, for instance, *Cavallo v. Star Enterprise.*[61] Mrs. Cavallo complained she was once, for a five-minute period, within 500 feet (presumably downwind) of an AvJet aviation fuel spill, and she attributed chronic health problems to the exposure she (and her symptomless husband) experienced. The court found no evidence of significant exposure or any correlation between her one-time exposure and her symptoms. The court noted, however:

> Also worth emphasizing is that the circumstances of each case are unique, and the absence of scientific validation through published studies and tested hypotheses is not always fatal to an expert's opinion. Specifically, there may be instances where the temporal connection between exposure to a given chemical and subsequent injury is so compelling as to dispense with the need for reliance on standard methods of toxicology.... For instance, if a known chemical is accidentally introduced into a company's ventilation system, and all of the workers exposed immediately develop the same adverse reaction, then the episode itself may be sufficiently indicative of causation.[62]

Where the opinions of the physicians are based upon standard methodologies, the *Frye/Daubert* analysis need not even be invoked:

> Here, the experts relied on air sampling, chemical analysis, examinations and questionnaires. These qualify as established scientific methods of the type relied upon by experts in the field, not novel scientific theories. Thus, we need not engage in a *Frye* analysis.[63]

The physician's taking of patient history, physical examination, and standard tests are not denigrated by the courts. Nor, for that matter, are specific epidemiological studies required. The insistence by defense experts upon double-blind, peer-reviewed, published studies of the precise exposures experienced by plaintiffs implies (incorrectly) that such information is required to be "scientific." Quite the contrary is true. In *Ferebee*, the Court of Appeals for the District of Columbia held:

> [A] cause-effect relationship need not be clearly established by animal or epidemiological studies before a doctor can testify that, in his opinion, such a relationship exists. As long as the basic methodology employed to reach such a conclusion is sound, such as the use of tissue samples, standard tests, and patient examination, products liability law does not preclude recovery until a "statistically significant" number of people have been injured or until science has had the time and resources to complete sophisticated laboratory studies of the chemical. In a courtroom, the test for allowing a plaintiff to recover in a tort suit of this type is not scientific certainty but legal sufficiency; if reasonable jurors *could* conclude from the expert testimony that paraquat more likely than not caused Ferebee's injury, the fact

that another jury might reach the opposite conclusion or that science would require more evidence before conclusively considering the causation question resolved is irrelevant. That Ferebee's case may have been the first of its exact type, or that his doctors may have been the first alert enough to recognize such a case, does not mean that the testimony of those doctors, who are concededly well qualified in their fields, should not have been admitted.

When we considered the all-important question of what evidence is *allowable* in a court of law to establish proximate cause (the cause-and-effect relationship between a toxic exposure and a given injury, for instance) we soon see that *Daubert* is the culmination of what had been a growing body of case law embracing a more sophisticated view of science than that articulated in *Frye v. United States.*[64]

In *Daubert I* (*Daubert* 1993), the Supreme Court recognized science as the product of the clash of competing theories which may be assessed by the jury on the merits — not as a body of dogma having "general acceptance" handed down from the scientific establishment, impervious to challenge by those outside.

> Nothing in the [Federal] Rules [of Evidence] as a whole or in the text and drafting history of Rule 702, which specifically governs expert testimony, gives any indication that "general acceptance" is a necessary precondition to the admissibility of scientific evidence. Moreover, such a rigid standard would be at odds with the Rules' liberal thrust and their general approach of relaxing the traditional barriers to "opinion" testimony.[65]

So long as a conclusion is reached through reasoning from scientific methods and tests, the fact that the conclusion may be controversial is not a basis for exclusion.

A trial judge determines the admissibility of evidence and the qualification of an expert to testify as a "preliminary question" in accordance with Federal Rule of Evidence 104(a). The Supreme Court in *Daubert I* called for a "preliminary assessment" of whether the testimony was "scientific knowledge" of assistance to the trier of fact.[66] The Third Circuit suggests restraint with respect to a trial court's conduct of this preliminary assessment:

> [The] judge should not exclude evidence simply because he or she thinks that there is a flaw in the expert's investigative process which renders the expert's opinions incorrect. The judge should only exclude evidence if the

flaw is large enough that the expert lacks "good grounds" for his or her conclusions.[67]

In *Daubert I*, the Supreme Court determined that the phrase "scientific knowledge" in Federal Rule of Evidence 702 establishes a standard of evidentiary reliability.[68] Is the expert proposing to testify to (1) scientific knowledge that (2) will assist the trier of fact to understand or determine a fact in issue? "This entails a *preliminary assessment* of whether the reasoning or methodology underlying the testimony is scientifically valid and of whether that reasoning or methodology properly can be applied to the facts in issue." (Emphasis added.)[69]

These are not truly rhetorical questions. They are intended to illustrate what the Ninth Circuit stated in *Daubert II*: "Something doesn't become 'scientific knowledge' just because it's uttered by a scientist; nor can an expert's self-serving assertion that his conclusions were 'derived by the scientific method' be deemed conclusive, else the Supreme Court's opinion [in *Daubert I*] could have ended with footnote two."[70]

Many plaintiffs' cases are based upon the conclusions reached by people trying to find answers: air test companies, treating physicians, fellow workers, family members. Such individuals are motivated to find answers. By contrast, it must be recalled that the defense experts have different motivations, which are oftentimes best served by a rigid and dogmatic adherence to orthodoxy — to what has been proven to a scientific certainty — even if it means that nothing is explained.

This is why *Daubert* came to be: to permit thoughtful, scientific analysis to be considered on its merits even if it lacked the imprimatur of the scientific establishment.

The debate is that science requires more than rigid orthodoxy in order to progress. It requires rigorous and constant reexamination in order to maintain its integrity. When the defense insists upon double-blind, peer-reviewed epidemiological studies before concluding that toxic fumes sicken workers, it is, for its own purposes, twisting scientific skepticism into caricature. The defense forgets science's thirst for problem-solving innovations. It dismisses the import of these eloquent words of Sir Bradford Hill:

> All scientific work is incomplete — whether it be observational or experimental. All scientific work is liable to be upset or modified by advancing knowledge. That does not confer upon us a freedom to ignore the knowledge we already have, or to postpone the action that it appears to demand at a given time.[71]

[82]

Multiple Chemical Sensitivity Syndrome

At the outset, we described a constellation of symptoms reported by workers. This constellation is increasingly gaining recognition within the medical community as Multiple Chemical Sensitivity Syndrome (MCSS). MCSS has been defined as "an acquired disorder characterized by recurrent symptoms, referable to multiple organ systems, occurring in response to demonstrable exposure to many chemically unrelated compounds at doses far below those established in the general population to cause harmful effects."[72] Across the country, numerous workers exposed to chemicals in the workplace have reported heightened sensitivity to low levels of chemicals at work and elsewhere, and report severe illness secondary to reexposure. In Canada, the Toronto Ministry of Health Report concluded:

> While we believe that there is evidence to support the view that a significant number of persons show symptoms of environmental hypersensitivity, we are unable to make any definitive statement about the prevalence of the disorder.[73]

The scientific uncertainty respecting toxic chemical exposures and the absence of any abnormal objective findings[74] in the worker reporting symptoms of MCSS impedes the treating physician in reaching a diagnosis of occupational disease. Physicians encountering the syndrome in isolated cases, lacking objective findings and finding standard medical treatment ineffective, have reacted with frustration, ascribing the symptoms to emotional disorders, often withdrawing their support from the patient.

In a recent report to the New Jersey Department of Health, the authors note:

> Acceptance of chemical sensitivity as *bona fide* physical disease may … be facilitated by the recognition that it is widespread in nature and is not limited to what some observers would describe as malingering workers, hysterical housewives, and workers experiencing mass psychogenic illness. We are struck by the fact that individuals in such demographically divergent groups as industrial workers, office workers, housewives, and children, report similar polysymptomatic complaints triggered by chemical exposures….
>
> Physicians who see more or less random individuals who are not members of an identifiable exposure group are less likely to recognize patterns or similarities among these patients who claim to be chemically sensitive….

[83]

> Once physicians recognize a constellation of symptoms that occur repeatedly in individuals who share similar exposure histories, the "disease" seems to change its label from "idiopathic" or "psychogenic" to a recognized disorder....[75]

Because *being believed* is of utmost importance to MCSS victims, the ability to obtain objective markers of toxic exposure becomes all the more important. Such markers may not show disease, but they may confirm that the symptoms of the patient are not fabricated, a confirmation that will help to earn the support of the treating doctor and the finder of fact, the jury.

Dr. Marks of the Department of Pharmacology and Toxicology, Faculty of Medicine, Queen's University, Kingston, Ontario, Canada, concluded that alterations of the heme biosynthetic pathway could be used as an index of exposure to a variety of toxic agents. In 1985, Dr. Marks wrote:

> The stage has now been reached where an understanding of the details of the heme biosynthetic pathway allows one to use alterations in this pathway as an index of exposure to a variety of toxic agents. The usefulness of the heme biosynthetic pathway as an indicator of exposure to toxic agents is due, at least in part, to the development in recent years of highly sensitive techniques to separate and measure porphyrins.[76]

Values on certain enzyme levels relating to the porphyrin byproducts of heme synthesis above the ninety-fifth percentile are usually evidence of disturbance of heme metabolism and can serve as a marker of toxic exposure.

MCSS exists, if not as a discrete disease, then as a clinically recognized constellation of symptoms. MCSS may not be "disproven" simply by disputes regarding its mechanism. The MCSS patient ought not to be evaluated or diminished by the "mechanism" of his or her ailment, whether it involves immunological, irritant, allergic, toxic, or psychological factors. The causation and manifestation of the ailment is likely to be multifactorial, interactive, and highly individual. That an autonomic irritant response supported by classical conditioning may account for some manifestations is not inconsistent with a toxic onset. Nor, for that matter, is evidence of derangement of metabolic function inconsistent with a psychologically mediated response. Biological systems, including human beings, are complex.

[84]

Other objective measures, such as SPECT scans and immunologic testing, may help piece together objective evidence. This evidence may help not only to establish the proximate cause needed by the courts, but to win the belief of the medical community, the lack of which has too often added insult to injury.

TORT PRINCIPLES AND WORKERS' COMPENSATION

It is important to acknowledge that the burden, however onerous, of establishing causation traditionally falls upon the plaintiff. For an injured worker, establishing a causal relationship between exposure to a novel chemical formulation and specific symptoms may constitute an insurmountable burden in the present environment of medical and scientific uncertainty, although recent shifts in the case authority will undoubtedly prove helpful. Poorly funded (often unemployed), sick, and desperate, workers suffering an occupational disease resulting from exposure to toxic chemicals in the workplace often are asked to establish, by a preponderance of the evidence (or more), the toxicity of chemicals whose effects have yet to be explored by the combined resources of industry, employer, or government agency, or to be generally recognized by the medical community.

The Washington Industrial Insurance Act (Workers' Compensation Act)[77] is based upon "a *quid pro quo* compromise between employees and employers"[78] in 1911: The employer consented to pay some claims for which it would not then have been liable under the common law in exchange for limited liability, and the employee gave up common law actions and remedies in exchange for "sure and certain relief." At the outset, the act provided basic coverage for injuries sustained in the course of employment, but specifically excluded coverage for disability resulting from occupational diseases. In 1937, the act was amended to provide compensation for disability or death caused by any one of 21 listed diseases. After a number of amendments in the intervening years, in 1961, the Legislature eliminated the list of compensable diseases and provided coverage for occupational diseases arising "naturally and proximately out of employment." When occupational diseases became compensable, the act became the exclusive remedy for employees against their employers for such diseases.[79]

The compensatory scheme has three basic elements: elimination of all civil actions against the employer; elimination of "fault" as an issue; and limitations on recovery of damages. In exchange the employees are to receive "sure and certain relief" and compensation for certain injuries that would have been barred by the common law of 1911.

The hope of "sure and certain relief" has proved illusory. In an occupational disease claim, the injured worker may, in fact, experience legal proceedings which are greater in number, duration, complexity, and expense than in the much criticized civil justice system.[80] The compensation for certain injuries barred by the common law of 1911 is scarcely less illusory: The common law at the turn of the nineteenth century was heavily tilted towards the employer through the availability of legal defenses such as contributory negligence, the "fellow servant" rule, and assumption of risk. In a finding of contributory negligence, the worker would be deprived of any recovery if negligent in *any* degree, regardless of the extent of the employer's negligence. The "fellow servant" doctrine denied any recovery to the worker if the injury had resulted in any degree from the negligence of a fellow worker. Finally, under assumption of risk, the worker could not recover any damages if the injury was due to an inherent hazard of the job that the worker should have had recognized in advance.

All of these rules have since been eliminated as prominent, operative features of the tort system. They were, in fact, transient alterations in the common law to encourage industrialization by making the burdens on industry as light as possible.[81]

> Dangerous enterprises, involving a high degree of risk to others, were clearly indispensable to the industrial and commercial development of a new country and it was considered that the interests of those in the vicinity of such enterprises must give way to them, and that too great a burden not be placed upon them. With the disappearance of the frontier, and the development of the country's resources, it was to be expected that the force of this objection would be weakened, and that it would be replaced in time by a view that the hazardous enterprise, even though it be socially valuable, must pay its way, and make good the damage inflicted.[82]

The workers' compensation system institutionalizes the relative power of industry and the worker at that historic interval in the early 1900s when the pendulum had swung to its extreme position of promoting industrial enterprise over individual rights, in the heyday of the railroad, before trade unions and the automobile. In short, the worker to this day labors under limitations in compensation in exchange for industry having yielded evanescent common law defenses about to be taken from it.

By contrast, the employer enjoys, under the Industrial Insurance Act, freedom from any civil action instituted by the worker even in cases of gross negligence. The principle establishing this act as the exclusive remedy for the injured worker yields only to actions against the employer for intentional injury (where the employer has the deliberate intention of producing such injury)[83] or for the tort of outrage (where the conduct is "so outrageous in character and so extreme in degree, as to go beyond all possible bounds of decency, and to be regarded as atrocious, and utterly intolerable in a civilized community").[84]

Two commentators reviewing a Florida case of two workers sexually assaulted and harassed by their supervisor on the job noted, with respect to workers' compensation laws similar to those in Washington:

> The suit was found barred by the exclusive remedy doctrine because the outrageous conduct of the supervisor could not be imputed to the employer. In its opinion, the court acknowledged that there would probably be no monetary recovery available under Workers' Compensation because the workers had not suffered any loss of wage-earning capacity. Nevertheless, the court held that the injuries arose out of the employment and were within the scope of Workers' Compensation. The exclusive remedy turned two multimillion dollar tort actions into two Workers' Compensation claims with recovery limited to actual medical expenses.[85]

Nowhere does the disparity between the civil justice system and the workers' compensation system loom larger than in the coverage for permanent disability. For loss of one eye by enucleation, the prescribed compensation as of this writing is $21,600; complete loss of hearing in one ear, $7,200; loss of all fingers except the thumb, $29,160; total bodily impairment, $90,000. Other unscheduled disabilities must be compared to percentage of total bodily impairment.[86] Death benefits are similarly limited: for a surviving spouse without children, 60 percent of the wages of the deceased worker, but not less than $185 per month, to cease upon remarriage. Burial expenses are not to exceed twice the monthly wage.[87]

The limitation on damages, accepted as central to the workers' compensation system, was recently rejected by the Washington State Supreme Court[88] in the context of civil actions as an intrusion into the province of the jury to determine damages. The effect of the limited recovery available to workers is to reduce incentive to uncover wrongdoing: Fault is not an issue. Limitations on damages discourage aggressive pursuit of the matter. Likewise, there is limited deterrence against wrongful conduct. The maximum exposure of the employer is limited, and the company has the resources and incentive to defend the case on the issues of causation.

We would not be surprised to learn that a corporate employer would decide whether to defend or pay a claim according to which presented the lesser expense. Entering into these calculations would be the expense associated with determining the risks of exposure and taking the ambitious industrial hygiene efforts needed to safeguard thousands of workers. The greater the limitation on damages, the more reduced the employer's economic incentive to eliminate the workplace exposure or take precautionary measures.

Self-insurers under the act, rather than contributing to the state fund for accident victims, have sufficient resources to themselves cover projected costs of injuries. This system gives the employer a direct financial stake in the outcome of each compensation claim. This economic sensitivity to outcome and concomitant desire to reduce overall costs, although presently encouraging the vigor of the defense on claims, may prove to be a valuable asset in restructuring the system to accomplish the policy goals articulated by Senator Reid years ago.

REDRESSING THE BALANCE

Modern tort analysis begins with the recognition that reasonable public conduct cannot be determined solely by assertion of private entitlements but depends, in part, upon policy decisions respecting cost avoidance. Oliver Wendell Holmes wrote: "If there is danger that harm to another will follow, the act is generally wrong in the eyes of the law."[89] This deceptively simple statement recognizes that the common law, outside of its historic commitment to the protection of private property rights, requires reasonable public conduct. Another noted jurist, Judge Learned Hand, held that the legal responsibility to avoid injuries to another was a function of the burden of preventative measures, the probability of injury and the gravity of the resulting injury, with liability arising if the burden of prevention is less than the product of the gravity of the resulting injury and the probability of its occurrence.[90]

It is immediately apparent that the "gravity" of the resulting injury is determined by dollars. Where, as in workers' compensation, the compensable value of injury is limited by schedule, the preventative measures reasonably undertaken by the employer based on economic factors will be similarly reduced, in effect lowering the requisite standard of care. If loss of hearing in one ear is worth $7,200 per worker, one could hardly expect protective measures significantly more costly than the compensable risk. Such risk to the employer may, in fact, be substantially offset if the costs of production are reduced by engaging in conduct which subjects workers to greater injury.[91]

The existing legal framework governing workers' compensation results in a misallocation of responsibility respecting the burden of establishing chemical toxicity. In effect, to establish causation, the worker is required to overcome a presumption of safety. If the worker fails to prove the harmfulness of the toxic exposure, the worker must bear the damages without assistance. As the standard of proof is rendered more rigorous, it becomes increasingly difficult for the worker to prevail. One author has noted that "requiring an epidemiologic standard of proof in these cases will essentially foreclose on the ability of many truly injured workers to recover any damages. The result will be to remove what apparently is one of the more potent driving forces behind workplace preventive measures."[92]

To redress the balance in favor of greater justice and reasonable accident avoidance, changes must be based upon well-established principles, starting first with the observation of Professor Calabresi: "What then are the principal goals of any system of accident law? First, it must be just or fair; second, it must reduce the costs of accidents."[93]

If the system requires injured workers to shoulder an evidentiary burden that the combined resources of government, industry, and the scientific and medical communities have been unable to meet, that system in effect allocates the cost of workplace injury to the worker. Public policy statements persuade us that this is not fair or just. More to the point, those best able to prevent injuries caused by toxic exposures are not encouraged to do so, while those powerless to avoid the injuries are largely uncompensated.

We have already seen that regulatory oversight sufficiently stringent to prevent toxic exposures is largely impracticable. There can be little doubt that the fines embodied in the Toxic Substances Control Act are insufficient to alter the incentives of the employer otherwise shielded from liability for the damages sustained by its workers. Moreover, increasing such fines, although a laudable suggestion, is unlikely to address with sufficient sensitivity the internal economic motivations of industry and employer. Instead, we must restructure the existing legal framework to maximize incentives for accident avoidance on the part of industry, employer, and worker, without reliance upon the creation of a massive regulatory and enforcement apparatus.

Historically, theories of liability and causation have both been modified when necessary to achieve justice. Strict liability, rather than negligence, has been applied to circumstances where people exposed to injury lacked sufficient knowledge to protect themselves: For example, unseaworthiness, a species of strict liability protecting seamen from defective conditions onboard ship, creates liability in the absence of negligence on the part of shipowners, in favor of seamen. Products liability is another example, protecting the user from product defects. Such allocations of liability recognize that "potential accident victims fear pain and suffering regardless of compensation, so they will be unaffected in their choices among acts and activities by our decision whether or not to compensate them."[94] Not only are the potentially injured parties fully motivated by the desire to avoid injury, but leaving their damages uncompensated cannot enhance motivation to avoid injury: They simply do not have enough knowledge to appreciate the risks arising from technology beyond obvious apprehension. The shipowners and manufacturers, regarded as having specialized knowledge, are held strictly liable for defects, which maximizes their incentive to design safe products and to design in anticipation of foreseeable product misuses. "The purpose of such [strict] liability is to insure that the costs of injuries resulting from defective products are borne by the manufacturers rather than by the injured persons who are powerless to protect themselves."[95]

The worker exposed to toxic chemicals has virtually no way of foreseeing the risks associated with exposure, and indeed, the risks may be largely unknown, as we have seen. Unlike the consumer, the employee even lacks the choice of refraining from product use. Leaving the risk of toxic injury on the worker, where the toxicology of the chemical is unknown, cannot reduce the cost of accidents. The three routes by which the worker may be protected are increased knowledge, product selection, and industrial hygiene measures; these are exclusively within the control of the manufacturer and employer. Both manufacturer and employer may respond to economic incentives to gain knowledge respecting the effects of toxic exposures from a given product; to disseminate such knowledge to workers; to implement workplace measures in the absence of complete knowledge; or to choose alternatives to the problematic product. The situation calls for strict liability. Such liability in the face of unprovable causation is a hollow remedy, however.

Traditional notions of causation have been modified in the past when justice so required. In *Sindell v. Abbott Laboratories*,[96] the court compromised traditional principles of causation by permitting liability based upon market share where over 200 companies had marketed the drug DES, implicated as a carcinogen, and the injured party had no way of discovering what manufacturer made the drug specifically administered to that party. In other words, establishing a strict causal relationship between a given plaintiff and a specific product or manufacturer was impossible — and held to be unnecessary.

There is precedent within the workers' compensation system to use presumptions to assist in establishing causation. For instance, under the Washington Industrial Insurance Act, there is a rebuttable presumption that respiratory disease is an occupational disease for firefighters.[97] Such a presumption for toxic exposures to workers for those symptoms identified in the material safety data sheets could address some of the impediments to establishing causation with minimal disruption to the existing compensatory scheme. Such a presumption, however, would not address the reduced motivation of employers to avoid workplace exposures as a result of the limitations on compensable damages. As it presently stands, even if the manufacturer provided the employer with complete toxicological information, the employer who routinely engaged in unsafe industrial hygiene practices in an effort to increase production or engaged in a program of product misuse could not be made to bear the full measure of damages resulting. Authorizing private civil actions by workers against employers for occupational diseases arising from toxic exposures would increase the worker's incentive to pursue litigation and heighten the risks the employer would face should the negligence continue. On the state level, the occupational disease coverage for toxic exposures could be withdrawn from the workers' compensation system. There was, after all, a time when no occupational diseases were covered by workers' compensation and a private civil action existed in its place.[98] Such an approach necessarily involves modification of the exclusive remedy provisions of the workers' compensation laws, which are central to the existing legislative scheme and which have been repeatedly and stringently upheld in Washington case authority.

In the alternative, on the federal level, a private right of action under TSCA, preempting state workers' compensation laws to the extent in conflict, could be authorized in addition to the present system of fines. Such an action could permit recovery of damages by workers for violations of TSCA, thereby easing the burden of its enforcement. Failure to comply with the industrial hygiene recommendations on the material safety data sheets could lead to the presumption of causation as to those symptoms reported on the MSDS.

Although these approaches will increase the employer's incentive to put protective measures into effect, they do not address the quantity or quality of information available to industry (upon which employers necessarily rely) because they do not motivate chemical manufacturers fully to develop toxicological data or to recommend stringent industrial hygiene measures in the absence of such data. Since toxicological data are likely to remain insufficient, we must determine who should bear the risk of the unknown consequences of exposure to unknown substances.

One of the hidden costs of the workers' compensation laws has been that, in the effort to obtain full compensation for injured workers, tort law has been stretched to expand third-party liability. Placing an affirmative duty on chemical manufacturers to assure adequate protective measures and training in the workplace would help prevent accidents. Such a duty, however, properly rests with the employer, and breach of that duty is more directly addressed by specific deterrence of wrongful acts by the employer. Nonetheless, accident avoidance would be furthered by a system in which chemical companies were required to communicate directly with the end users to assure that hazards are understood.

Without any alteration in the workers' compensation act, strict liability of chemical companies for injuries arising from toxic exposures could be restructured to place the burden of injury on the manufacturer, as the party best able to avoid the social cost of toxic exposures by thorough investigation, as well as to spread such costs by passing the expense of research and development through to its customers. Existing Washington law already creates strict liability for product manufacturers.[99] Moreover, enacted limitations on joint and several liability among joint tortfeasors arguably do not extend to cases involving hazardous substances.[100]

Modification of the existing Washington Products Liability statute could enhance worker safety. Generally, manufacturers have been permitted to interpose defenses of "state of the art" and "product misuse." These defenses generally preclude recovery where the product is made to the highest standard presently known or has not been used as intended. Neither defense should apply against a worker injured by exposure to a toxic chemical. Toxic chemicals clearly may prove hazardous even if made to the highest level of present technology, and workers clearly have no say as to how a product is used.

Adverse health effects from exposure to "space age" chemicals and composites ought to be presumed, with the chemical manufacturer held strictly liable for such an "ultrahazardous" product. The chemical manufacturer, however, should have a claim against the employer if its product is misused or if the specifications required by the employer are such that even with "state of the art" manufacture, the product cannot be handled safely. The employer should be able to assert the defense of product defect: A product should be considered defective if its MSDS and labelling do not include specific industrial hygiene measures capable of eliminating any foreseeable adverse health effects of exposure. The claim by the manufacturer against the employer for product misuse, however, would be established if it were determined that the employer failed to institute the industrial hygiene requirements identified by the manufacturer, requirements but for which the worker would not have been injured. An employer found liable should forfeit recovery on any workers' compensation lien for employee benefits paid.

Where an employee sues a third party such as a chemical company and that company, in turn, seeks recovery against the employer, it is termed a "third-party-over" case.[101] Such cases have been held to circumvent the exclusive remedy provisions of the Industrial Insurance Act on the grounds that the act "immunizes" the employer from any liability arising from a workplace injury; the Washington Supreme Court held that legislative action would be required to permit a third party to receive contribution from the employer in the absence of an independent duty between the third party and the employer in the form of a written indemnification agreement.[102] The Legislature should act.

Streamlining claims of workers against chemical manufacturers, and in turn permitting third-party-over claims by the chemical manufacturer against the employer, would maximize the utility of the MSDS. The chemical manufacturer could recoup any damages paid to the worker, for even unknown adverse effects, by requiring industrial hygiene practices calculated to address the risk and establishing the employer's failure to comply with them. The employer, in turn, would have incentives to comply fully with the MSDS requirements of workplace protection. Such a scheme would prevent the workers' compensation laws, intended as a shield for the workers, from being used as a shield from liability by the negligent employer who subjects the workers to risks (and profits thereby).

So long as the existing compensatory regime fails to maximize incentives for workplace safety, it unwittingly assures that the workplace will remain a "test tube" and the workers "guinea pigs." At present, the worker injured by toxic chemical exposure, which the worker is powerless to prevent, must submit to a punishing and tortuous procedure requiring a standard of proof that has eluded the grasp of employer, industry, government, science and medicine — or else go uncompensated. As Oliver Wendell Holmes put it, "A law which punished conduct which would not be blameworthy in the average member of the community would be too severe for that community to bear."[103] Such is the case here.

POST SCRIPT

In a unanimous 9–0 decision filed October 1995 in the case of *Birklid v. Boeing,* the Washington State Supreme Court, for the first time since 1922, found enough evidence to permit the question of an employer's "deliberate intention" to injure its workers to go to a jury. An injury inflicted upon a worker deliberately has always been an exception to worker's compensation permitting a direct claim against the employer. In *Birklid v. Boeing,* the State Supreme Court found that "actual knowledge" of "certain injury" and "willfully disregarding" that knowledge could constitute such deliberate intention to cause injury. The Court held, in its concluding sentence: "the blood of the worker" being "a cost of production ... no longer reflects the public policy or the law of Washington."

In *Birklid v. Boeing,* fourteen workers, supported by sworn statements and documents obtained from Boeing during nearly ten years of litigation, showed that Boeing knowingly exposed workers to toxic substances in the form of phenol formaldehyde impregnated materials (phenolic prepregs), knowing that they would be injured. In spring and summer 1987, during material research and development, an internal Boeing memorandum, after describing innumerable symptoms reported by workers including dizziness, burning eyes, and upset stomachs, stated: "We anticipate this problem to increase as temperatures rise and production increases." The following month, the request for ventilation was denied, stating: "The odor level of the phenolic prepregs relative to other materials currently used ... does not warrant expenditure of funds for additional ventilation at this time." The material was introduced into full-scale production in August 1987. The building was freezing in the winter and, during summer months, temperatures rose to over 110 degrees. Nearly a dozen affidavits attested to workplace conditions being dramatically changed in advance of air monitoring by government agencies: cleanup was commenced, operations cut back, doors were opened, and fans brought in — just to be removed following testing. Rather than correcting the harm, the evidence offered by dozens of witnesses demonstrated a pattern of stifling worker reports of injury including discouraging the reporting of symptoms. The suit also included claims that human "experiments" had been conducted — exposing workers to chemicals while being monitored and causing them to react with violent nausea and vomiting.

Following the Supreme Court decision, Boeing and other employers lobbied the legislature to change the law so that an employer would not be liable even if it knowingly injured workers — so long as the injury occurred while advancing a business purpose. This was the same argument Boeing had advanced in the State Supreme Court unsuccessfully. After passing the State Senate, the proposed legislation was rejected by the State House in a dramatic vote involving no fewer than eight votes changing at the last minute.

Just weeks before a trial was to commence in the United States District Court in June 1997, the case was settled for an undisclosed amount. It had been ten years since the workers had first been exposed to the toxic chemicals.

References

1. S. Hrg. 101–112, "Issues Related to the Use of, and Exposure to, Various Chemicals," Hearings Before the Subcommittee on Toxic Substances, Environmental Oversight, Research and Development of the Committee on Environment and Public Works, United States Senate, March 6, 1989 (Washington: 1989).

2. S. Hrg. 101–112, p. 6.

3. S. Hrg. 101–112, pp. 55–57, 268–80.

4. S. Hrg. 101–112, pp. 56–57.

5. *See* Occupational Safety and Health Act, 29 U.S.C. Sec. 651 (1976).

6. S. Hrg. 101–112, p. 277.

7. 15 U.S.C. §§ 2601–2629 (1982).

8. S. Hrg. 101–112, pp. 235–36, 240.

9. S. Hrg. 101–112, pp. 260–61.

10. S. Hrg. 101–112, p. 266.

11. M. S. Breysse, "Industrial Hygiene Problems Associated with Recognition and Assessment of Exposure to Composites," *Applied Industrial Hygiene* (December 1989): 81–82.

12. S. E. Feinman, *Formaldehyde Sensitivity and Toxicity* (Boca Raton, Fla.: CRC, 1988), p. 28.

13. Breysse, p. 82, citing M. Bruze, "Contact Sensitizers in Resins Based on Phenol and Formaldehyde," *Acta Dermato-Venereologica Supplement 119* (1985), writes: "Researchers in Sweden reported isolating a number of contact sensitizers in resins based on phenol formaldehyde. Prior to this series of studies, only 4 sensitizers were recognized in phenol formaldehyde compounds including 2-methyl phenol, 4-methol phenol, 2, 3, 6-trimethyl phenol, and formaldehyde. Utilizing guinea pigs and humans, 11 new contact sensitizers were isolated; however, this study did not examine the possible effects of respiratory exposures."

14. S. A. Roach and S. M. Rappaport, "But They Are Not Thresholds: A Critical Analysis of the Documentation of Threshold Limit Values," *American Journal of Industrial Medicine* 17 (1990): 727–53.

15. Roach and Rappaport, p. 729, citing ACGIH, "Threshold Limit Values and Biological Exposure Indices for 1988–89" (Cincinnati, Ohio: American Conference of Governmental Industrial Hygienists, 1988).

16. Roach and Rappaport, p. 732.

17. Roach and Rappaport, p. 732.

18. Roach and Rappaport, p. 742.

19. Castleman and Ziem, "Corporate Influence on Threshold Limit Values," *American Journal of Industrial Medicine* 13 (1988): 531–59.

20. Castleman and Ziem, p. 531.

21. Castleman and Ziem, p. 556.

22. RCW 51.28.055 provides, in pertinent part, that: "Claims for occupational disease or infection to be valid and compensable must be filed within two years following the date the worker had written notice from a physician: (1) Of the existence of his or her occupational disease, and (2) That a claim for disability benefits may be filed."

23. Green, "The Paradox of Statutes of Limitations in Toxic Substance Litigation," *California Law Review* 76 (October 1988): 965.

24. Irving J. Selikoff, Keynote Address to "Occupational Health in the 1990s," *Annals of the New York Academy of Sciences* 572 (1989): 4.

25. As technology currently stands, approximation and analogy are the imperfect tools available to expedite chemical testing. The EPA employs what it terms "structure activity relationships" (SAR) and "quantitative structure activity relationships" (QSAR) as screening tools to help determine which new chemicals need to be controlled or screened. This approach involves review of existing data; analogy with data available on other related chemicals; mathematical expressions for biological activity; scientific judgment and assessment. Computer modeling, if advanced to the stage where human toxicological response could be determined without being limited by the ethical and time constraints, to which human experimentation is subject, could accelerate testing. The

necessary database for such a program would undoubtedly be the crowning success of a biotechnology far ahead of anything foreseeable for decades.

26. Richard S. Cornfeld, and Michael B. Minton, "How to Defend Against an Adverse Epidemiological Study," *BNA Toxics Law Reporter*, February 8, 1989, p. 1092.

27. "Compensating Victims of Pollution: The Workers' Compensation Experience." Statement of Leslie I. Boden, Assistant Professor of Economics, Occupational Health Program and Department of Health Policy and Management, Harvard School of Public Health, Before the Subcommittee on Commerce, Transportation and Tourism of the Committee on Energy and Commerce, U.S. House of Representatives, November 22, 1983, at 6 [original emphasis].

28. Dore, "A Commentary on the Use of Epidemiological Evidence in Demonstrating Cause-in-Fact," *Harvard Environmental Law Review* 7 (1983): 429, 434.

29. 736 F.2d 1529, 1535–36 (D.C. Cir.), *cert. denied*, 469 U.S. 1062 (1984).

30. The "dose-response" relationship, which correlates extent of exposure with certain symptoms, requires precise knowledge of test techniques to determine the exposure (dermal, inhalation of vapors, particulate exposures, ingestion), it is important to recognize that "air test levels" are useless for testing routes of exposure other than respiration of vapors. It is often impossible to determine the total individual exposure. Permissible exposure limits established by the government rely heavily upon studies conducted upon white males based upon an eight-hour workday; consequently, even these guidelines for the "average" worker may not be instructive for a wide variety of workers who differ from the study cohorts by virtue of body size, gender, other characteristics relevant to physiological response, or length of workday.

31. *Brock v. Merrell Dow Pharmaceuticals, Inc.*, 874 F.2d 307 (5th Cir. 1989); *Heyman v. United States*, 506 F. Supp. 1145, 1149 (S. D. Fla. 1981). ("Given the general inability of a physician to make accurate predictions of causation without at least some reference to epidemiological studies, plaintiff's position that her illness was caused by the swine flu shot amounts to nothing more than speculation.")

32. *See, e.g.* Nace, "Standard of Proof in Drug and Toxic Tort Products Liability Cases — 'Preponderence' or 'Scientific Certainty'," *Products Liability Law Journal* 1 (October 1988): 87; Cheek, "Legal vs. Medical Criteria for Determining Causation in Occupational Disease Claims," *Annals of the New York Academy of Sciences* 572 (1989): 17.

33. NIOSH *Current Intelligence Bulletin* 50 (August 1988): 2. (Quoted in Breysse, *op. cit.*, App. E.)

34. Id. at 25.

35. *Ferebee*, 1529, 1536.

36. 113 S. Ct. 2786 (1993).

37. Rule 702 provides: "If scientific, technical, or other specialized knowledge will assist the trier of fact to understand the evidence or to determine a fact in issue, a witness qualified as an expert by knowledge, skill, experience, training, or education, may testify thereto in the form of an opinion or otherwise."

38. 66 Wn. App. 644, 661–62 (1992).

39. At 1535.

40. 77 Wn. App. 201, 216 (1995).

41. *See also Osburn v. Anchor Labs, Inc.*, 825 F.2d 908, 914–915 (5th Cir. 1987) (an expert physician's opinion on causation need not be generally accepted in the scientific community; it is the *methods* upon which the expert relies in forming his or her opinion that must be generally accepted), *cert. denied*, 485 U.S. 1009 (1988).

42. *Intalco* at 654; *Hamilton v. Dep't of Labor & Industries*, 11 Wn.2d 569, 571 (1988).

43. *Intalco* at 657–58.

44. *Intalco* at 663–64.

45. Such a case is *Grimes v. Hoffmann-LaRoche*, 907 F. Supp. 33 (D.N.H. 1995), in which the issue was whether cataracts could be caused by prescription doses of Accutane. Such a claim necessarily depends upon expert epidemiological testimony to establish causation.

46. 304 U.S. 64 (1938).

47. *Bruns* at 205.

48. *Bruns* at 205.

49. *Bruns* at 207.

50. *Bruns* at 207.

51. *Bruns* at 211–12.

52. *Bruns* at 213.

53. *Bruns* at 217.

54. Under Washington law, even with respect to medical issues, when the results of an alleged act of negligence are within the experience and observation of an ordinary lay person, the trier of fact can draw a conclusion as to the causal link without resort to expert testimony. *Riggins v. Bechtel Power Corp.*, 44 Wn. App. 244, 254, 722 P.2d 819 (1986); *Bennett v. Department of Labor & Industries*, 95 Wn.2d 531, 533, 627 P.2d 104 (1981); *Sacred Heart Medical Center v. Carrado*, 92 Wn.2d 631, 600 P.2d 1015 (1979).

55. The Court of Appeals in *Bruns*, 77 Wn. App. at 212, refused to distinguish *Intalco* as dealing with workplace conditions rather than design defects as urged by the defense holding.

56. *Intalco*, at 660.

57. 115 Idaho 1087, 1095, 772 P.2d 725 (Ct. App. 1989).

58. *Daubert v. Merrell Dow Pharmaceuticals, Inc.*, 43 F. 3d 1311 (9th Circuit), *cert. denied*, 116 S. Ct. 189 (1995).

59. *Daubert* (1995) at 1314.

60. It must be recalled that the air testing conducted by the defense will often fail to replicate the conditions of exposure either because of the alteration of conditions or the passage of time. This must be likened to testing the "reverse" side of the plate in the investigation of food poisoning.

61. 892 F. Supp. 756 (1995).

62. *Cavallo* at 773–74.

63. *Bruns* at 216.

64. 293 F. 1013 (D.C. Cir. 1923). See *Ferebee*; *Osburn v. Anchor Labs, Inc.*, 825 F. 2d 908, 914–15 (5th Cir. 1987) *cert. denied*, 485 U.S. 1009 (1988); and *Intalco*.

65. *Daubert* (1993) at 2790.

66. *Daubert* (1993) at 2796.

67. *Paoli R.R. Yard PCB Litigation*, 35 F.3d 717, 746 (1994).

68. *Daubert* (1993) at 2796.

69. *Daubert* (1993) at 2796.

70. *Daubert* (1995) at 1315–16.

71. A. B. Hill, "The Environment and Disease: Association or Causation?" *Proceedings of the Royal Society of Medicine* 58 (1965): 295–300.

72. Mark R. Cullen, "The Worker with Multiple Chemical Sensitivities: An Overview," *Occupational Medicine: State of the Art Reviews* 2, no. 2 (October-December 1987): 655, 657.

73. "Report of the Ad Hoc Committee on Environmental Hypersensitivity Disorders," Office of the Minister of Health, Toronto, Canada, 1985, p. 233.

74. "Report of the Ad Hoc Committee," p. 18; Cullen, p. 657.

75. Ashford and Miller, "Chemical Sensitivity: A Report to the New Jersey State Department of Health," December 1989, pp. ii–iv, 13.

76. G. S. Marks, "Exposure to Toxic Agents: The Heme Biosynthetic Pathway and Hemoproteins as Indicator," *CRC Critical Reviews in Toxicology* 15, no. 2 (1985): 151.

77. RCW 51.04.010 *et seq.*

78. *Wolf v. Scott Wetzel Services*, 113 Wn.2d 665, 668 (1989); *McCarthy v. Department of Social and Health Services*, 110 Wn.2d 812, 816 (1988); *Sterz v. Industrial Insurance Commission*, 91 Wash. 588, 590 (1916).

79. *McCarthy*, at 816; RCW 51.16.16.040; RCW 51.32.180.

80. In a recent lead poisoning case, the author undertook representation of the worker in 1989 just prior to the commencement of trial before the Board of Industrial Insurance Appeals. The worker had been poisoned between 1980 and 1984. The board reversed the determination of the Department of Labor and Industries denying the existence of an occupational disease. Such a result may be appealed to a *de novo* trial before the Superior Court jury on the transcript (RCW 51.52.115). After exhaustion of all appeals through the judicial system, if the finding of the board reversing the department's order is upheld, the matter will be remanded to the department for determination of the extent of disability and appropriate compensation. The jurisdiction of the board on appeal is limited to the scope of the department order denying the existence of an occupational disease (*Lenk v. Department of Labor and Industries*, 3 Wn. App. 977, 982 [1970]). The department's determination of disability will then be subject to repetition of the appellate review outlined above. In the civil justice system, determination of both liability and damages would occur simultaneously in a single proceeding.

81. M. Horwitz, *The Transformation of American Law 1780–1860* (Cambridge, Mass.: Harvard University Press, 1977). For instance, in the early nineteenth century it was accepted that the master was responsible to all injured parties for the acts of his servant.

82. Prosser, *Law of Torts*, 4th edition (St. Paul: 1971), at 509.

83. RCW 51.24.020; *See Foster v. Allsop Automatic, Inc.*, 86 Wn.2d 579, 584 (1976).

84. *Guffey v. State*, 103 Wn.2d 144, 146 (1984), quoting *Grimsby v. Samson*, 85 Wn.2d 52, 59 (1975). *See also Wolf v. Scott Wetzel Services*, 113 Wn.2d 665, 678 (1989).

85. DeCarlo and Minkowitz, "Workers' Compensation and Employers' Liability Law: National Developments and Trends," *Zippy Mart, Inc.*, 470 So.2d 720 (Fla. Dist. Ct. App. 1985).

86. RCW 51.32.080.

87. RCW 51.32.050.

88. *Sofie vs. Fibreboard Corp.*, 112 Wn.2d 636 (1989).

89. Holmes, *The Common Law* (Boston: 1881, 1923), p. 162.

90. *United States v. Carroll Towing Company*, 159 F.2d 169 (2d Cir. 1947).

91. On an individual level, it is the equivalent of a driver choosing to drive without a pollution control device where the use of such a device reduces gas mileage 30 percent, the fine is only $50, and the chance of citation is small.

92. Ozonoff, "Medical and Legal Causation," *Annals of the New York Academy of Sciences* 572 (1989): 23, 25.

93. G. Calabresi, *The Costs of Accidents: A Legal and Economic Analysis* (New Haven and London: Yale University Press, 1970), p. 24.

94. Calabresi, p. 22, n. 5.

95. *Greenman v. Yuba Power Products, Inc.,* 59 Cal.2d 67, 27 Cal. Rptr. 697, 377 P.12d 897 (Cal. 1963).

96. 607 P.2d 924 (Cal. 1980).

97. RCW 51.32.185.

98. *McCarthy v. Department of Social and Health Services,* 110 Wn.2d 812, 817 (1988); *Pellerin v. Washington Veneer Co.,* 163 Wash. 555, 558–59 (1931); *Depre v. Pacific Coast Forge Col,* 145 Wash. 263, 264 (1927).

99. RCW 7.72.030.

100. RCW 4.22.070(3)(a) provides: "Nothing in this section affects any cause of action relating to hazardous wastes or substances or solid waste disposal sites."

101. DeCarlo and Minkowitz, pp. 522–23.

102. *Glass v. Stahl Specialty Co.,* 97 Wn.2d 880 (1982); *Jones v. Robert E. Bayley Construction Co.,* 36 Wn. App. 357 (1984).

103. Holmes, p. 50.

III

SCIENCE AND
THE LITERATURE

That the pen is mightier than the sword has long been a given. Because some factions have virtually declared war on open recognition of the injuries caused by low levels of toxic chemicals, it is advantageous to spend some time examining the literature.

This literature has done much to add insult to real chemical injury. Essentially the view is that the symptoms of chemical sensitivity are a cry from people who have psychogenic illnesses and want a free lunch. In no case have the individuals who put out such nonsense ever run appropriate tests or performed objective studies of the chemically injured. Nevertheless, the literature is full of material used with a vengeance to "prove" that taking these people seriously is a disservice to the taxpayer and a needless scare to the rest of the population.

Chapter 6 provides an overview of the scientific method — real science as opposed to junk — and its importance in evaluating the literature on MCS. Chapter 7 examines some of the literature often cited by those opposed to any program recognizing the physiological effects of low levels of toxic exposure.

6. JUNK SCIENCE

Bonnye Matthews

A few years ago a new term appeared, "junk science." Books have appeared on the topic. The Internet is full of discussions on the subject, led by persons proclaiming themselves to be experts. But "junk science" is an oxymoron, a meaningless buzzword that only hinders understanding and communication. "Science," according to the dictionary, is "knowledge covering general truths or the operation of general laws especially as obtained and tested through the scientific method." If the research method is scientific, the result may be regarded as science. Research by other methods produces junk. Junk and science are mutually exclusive.

THE SCIENTIFIC METHOD AND ITS SAFEGUARDS

The scientific method is the way that most scientists since Galileo in the 1600s have approached their problem-solving efforts. Here are the basic steps:

1. **Starting point:** Identify a problem, question, or desire to know why something works or does not work.
2. **Objective:** Define the problem so that the goal of the research or experiment is clear.
3. **Study:** Gather data, read, ask questions.
4. **Consider alternatives:** Think about all the possible solutions to the problem.
5. **Develop hypothesis:** From available facts, decide which is the most likely to solve the problem (the chosen one is called the *hypothesis*).

6. **Check hypothesis:** Set up experiment to test the hypothesis; reproduce the experiment to determine whether the results are consistent.

Some considerations for setting up experiments are having *large numbers* of subjects to test (data on just a few subjects could skew results); controlling *variables* (eliminating factors that could affect individual results, such as temperature, humidity, time of day, differences in testing procedures); and adhering to *ethics* (for example, if subjects are human, could the experiment harm?).

7. **Test validity:** Compare results to hypothesis. If the experiment was properly set up, and results are inconsistent with hypothesis, the hypothesis is incorrect (not valid) and another solution must be examined.

8. **Test reliability:** Compare results to results; look at the data from each time the experiment was performed. If the experiment does not work out each time it is tried, the hypothesis is incorrect (not reliable) and another solution must be examined.

9. **Develop conclusion:** Once the experiment shows both validity and reliability, the conclusion can be drawn; that conclusion becomes a theory.

10. **Learn:** Remember the theory so that it may facilitate future problem-solving, while keeping an open mind that though the conclusion looks right, it may be dead wrong.

The ten steps seem so simple. As long as the scientist is unbiased and unfettered in his or her pursuit of fact, the process can be effective and efficient. The minute the funding source of a scientific pursuit has any interest in the outcome, science ceases to be science. It isn't "junk science"; it is just junk.

To further confuse the picture, it is possible to set up an experiment that appears to "prove" a hypothesis when just the reverse is true. Just because the numbers add a certain way, a conclusion is not necessarily valid. Anyone with a smattering of statistics knows that numbers can be manipulated to show what one wishes to show. This sort of manipulation is not limited to medical research. It takes place anytime the objective becomes to convince.

There are controls and safeguards that attempt to prevent such corruption of research. One is the process of "peer review." Peer review means that scientists in the same discipline review the work of the authors and provide their evaluation of the work. Unfortunately, there is bias in the peer review process.

Some medical journals, for example, consider themselves peer-reviewed. What that may mean at the very least is that *some* of the articles in an issue run through a peer review process; others don't. One key to the potential for bias in medical journal material is the list of the journal's directors and the financial base of the publication. Some corporations will offer journals free peer review by their employed scientists. Although some of these free reviewers may provide scientific assessments, there is so much room for conflict of interest that bias should be suspected.

A common corruption often missed totally by the peer review process is "mutual attribution." Here's how it works. Let's say I've done a study and found that my hypothesis appears to be valid. I write up my study and send it to others for review. I send it to people who I think will have a positive reaction to it — and they do. They even quote it in articles they are authoring. Now, I set about to write my next paper on the same subject. I quote my article and the ones written by the colleagues who have quoted my paper. This is mutual attribution. We do this as long as we write on the same subject. Within a short time, a few of us have developed a significant body of literature on the subject. Because the lead author's name shifts from one article to another, it appears that many of us have independently come to the same conclusions. Our material is published in respected journals. The data may be incorrect, but that is no longer an issue. Our medical opinion is well entrenched and there are numbers of sound financial resources urging more research. We gain respect — even if what we publish is junk.

Medical journals have another control: the letters written to the journal after an article is published. The journal management decides whether to publish. Once again, bias on the part of the journal's directors or financial backers can play a part in the decision. By failing to publish dissenting voices, a journal can perpetuate the illusion that no dissent exists.

EPIDEMIOLOGY

Proper examination is difficult in what might be considered pure science. When the experimentation involves human subjects, that level of difficulty increases. The study of life factors and how they relate to human health is called *epidemiology*. It is an imprecise field of inquiry. Scientists know that. An article in a medical journal, particularly an article involving a new area of study, is generally given a wait-and-see response. For a study to be valid, large numbers of subjects must be involved. It is impractical, if not utterly unethical, to assemble thousands of individuals and test whether a new medication has harmful effects on them. Epidemiology, nevertheless, is designed to study life factors and their relationship to human health and from that to develop the relative risk of developing a health problem from a certain life factor. By gathering data on thousands of individuals, epidemiologists then generate what they hope is statistically valid data for a population. With statistics, a rule is that generalized data cannot be ascribed to the individual. For example, wearing a safety helmet while riding a bicycle does not guarantee that a particular child will *not* experience brain damage in a bicycle crash, any more than failing to wear one guarantees damage in a bicycle crash.

Epidemiology is an inexact science. It is not possible to control variables. It is hoped that large numbers will smooth out the effect of variables. Other factors believed to enhance epidemiological validity are the credentials of those doing the research and the respect afforded the journal publishing the research. Other questions to ask, in evaluating the data, include the following: Are the populations properly selected? Has the same study been replicated by scientists unaffiliated with the reporting group? Is the conclusion (hypothesis) valid, or is an unknown factor influencing the results? Are results consistent with overall research? (If not, which is wrong?) Even with all these factors appearing to be carefully designed and controlled, there may still be problems.

Epidemiology has a use that seems to have escaped public notice. Decisions made by governmental officials are often based on epidemiological conclusions. The effect can be incredibly significant. It can also be incredibly irresponsible.

MEDICINE TODAY:
FOLLY WITHOUT A FAIL-SAFE SWITCH

Before one country actually proceeds to drop a bomb on another country, there are — one hopes — processes and procedures to assure that the action is taken only under a tightly prescribed set of circumstances. Such is not the case with medical science. For example, there is no mechanism for a doctor to reverse his or her own opinion. Why this is so defies comprehension. The danger is that such a view easily leads doctors to think themselves infallible. It leads to arrogance. If a doctor's opinion is in keeping with standard medical thought at the time, it's viewed as right, despite the fact that it may be dead wrong. Such a view leaves those best equipped to practice medical science in a box where delusion is a real hazard. Rather than face scorn for a change of view, doctors may do all manner of things to maintain an expressed opinion — even when they know better. There is peer pressure to do so. To do otherwise is to invite insult and lose respect.

Under the current structure of the development of medical literature, to assume that peer review is a safeguard is folly, to assume that respected journals publish legitimate articles is folly, to assume that universities publish material of better quality than other organizations is folly, to assume that credentials impart trustability is folly, to assume that bias is bridled and that science is not trash just because it looks that way is folly. To assume that numbers in epidemiology amount to anything more than a good guess is folly. To rest one's conviction on epidemiology, with its manipulable numbers, is folly.

Yet it is just this folly that the chemically injured face. The courts for cases in litigation believe in the validity of articles from peer-reviewed journals, even when those articles are patently trash. On top of this problem, the chemically injured also face accusations and assault from self-proclaimed experts outside of the medical establishment. In January 1997, John Stossel of the ABC television news program *20/20* did a piece on "junk science" — that oxymoron again! — in which he made it appear that he sees the chemically injured as pathetic psychiatric cases. Author Peter Huber, in his *Phantom Risk* (MIT Press, 1993), states, "Medical scientists have been unable to identify any specific physiological condition associated with MCS." By 1993, however, it was clear that toxic encephalopathy and other neuropathies were characteristic of cases of disabling MCS. Folly abounds, and the chemically injured suffer.

[107]

The structure of medical practice is changing also, though the change is slower than the shifts in literature. Perhaps this is nothing but a reflection of the entire discipline of medical science. Group medical practice, for example, has made significant changes in the way patients are approached. A most significant aspect of most of the new plans is the establishment of a gatekeeper. A gatekeeper essentially decides who will receive medical care and who will not. Many patients have recently discovered the changes that a shift to group practice has made. Their complaints fall into the dead spaces of air between patients garbaged in and out of an unimaginative system. Patients with chemical injury whose insurance coverage is tied to group medical clinic plans routinely are swept away by gatekeepers. When bottom lines drive science, bad medicine is one result.

THE FALLACY OF "INTRINSIC" KNOWLEDGE

Rather than use the strict trial by science which most scientists would ascribe to, medicine today is relying heavily on trial by Hippocratic method, while at the same time the Hippocratic oath has fallen into disuse. Hippocrates believed that intrinsic knowledge leads to truth in medicine. That truth was not to be questioned by a nonphysician. Intrinsic knowledge supposedly lies within the physician; it is dependent upon social position and social understanding, not biologic fact or reality. It is the stuff of which delusions are made. This type of "knowledge" is protected as a religious fanatic protects the beliefs of his cult. Because an intrinsic belief is part of a person's essential makeup, questioning that belief represents destruction of the person. Whether in medicine or any other field, anyone would resist such questioning with the utmost ferocity. And so the physician's view is accepted as if it had come from a god, partly due to societal conditioning and partly due to failure to question. Acceptance is all the more enthusiastic when the doctor says what one wishes to hear.

Scientific theories are observations of apparent truths — descriptions of a perceived reality. They are not reality in and of themselves. Many scientific theories fail to withstand the test of time. They are then replaced by other theories based on new data or better understanding of the subject under discussion.

Many of today's medical researchers — at least those currently being published — seem to have manufactured their science to fit preconceived notions of what multiple chemical sensitivity or injury is. Their papers appear more concerned with the impression that it was social and political science that fits the demands of the moment than with pragmatic and truthful science that advances the practice of medicine. In the following chapter, their work will be examined to determine whether it truly represents the scientific information that has accumulated regarding multiple chemical sensitivity or injury.

Research produces science when it is conducted in a manner consistent with the rules of science. Anything inconsistent with those rules is junk. In our modern age, we can have as much disinformation as information. No longer is it safe, if it ever has been, to trust that "professionals" behave professionally. It is incumbent upon the individual to take responsibility for himself: to be informed, to refuse to accept what anyone would have him believe without testing for himself, to trust only those he carefully deems worthy of trust.

Anyone with a strong desire for knowledge can evaluate the literature for himself. The standard against which any article must be judged is the scientific method. It must be kept in mind that even so, when a professional writes, you will not be privy to the raw data. All you can really do is determine whether the material withstands scrutiny according to the scientific method. Using this touchstone, however, you may be amazed to discover that much of what's out there is nothing but junk.

7. MEDICAL LITERATURE AND MCS: AN ANALYSIS OF SEVEN PAPERS

Donald L. Dudley, M.D.

In a focus on multiple chemical sensitivity seven authors collaborated to produce a two-part article published in the *Journal of Occupational Medicine* (1994; 36:718–730 and 731–737). This article was purported to provide significant findings regarding multiple chemical sensitivity. The title of the article is "Multiple Chemical Sensitivity Syndrome: A Clinical Perspective. I. Case Definition, Theories of Pathogenesis, and Research Needs. II. Evaluation, Diagnostic Testing, Treatment, and Social Considerations." The authors are P. J. Sparks, W. Daniell, D. W. Black, H. M. Kipen, L. E. Altman, G. E. Simon, and A. I. Terr.

MATERIAL

In my attempt to understand the conclusions of the two-part article, I chose to review seven papers written previously by the authors and referred to in their text and bibliography. My goal was to determine whether the previous articles were science. The articles I chose were

Sparks, P. J., G. E. Simon, W. J. Katon, L. C. Altman, G. H. Ayars, and R. L. Johnson: "An outbreak of illness among aerospace workers." *Western Journal of Medicine*, 1990; 153:28–33.
Simon, G. E., W. Daniell, H. Stockbridge, K. Claypoole, and L.

Rosenstock: "Immunologic, psychological, neuropsychological factors in multiple chemical sensitivity." *Annals of Internal Medicine,* 1993; 119:97–103.

L. C. Grammer, K. E. Harris, M. A. Shaughnessy, P. Sparks, G. H. Ayars, and R. Patterson: "Clinical and immunologic evaluation of 37 workers exposed to gaseous formaldehyde." *Journal of Allergy and Clinical Immunology,* 1990; 86:177–181.

Black, D. W., A. Rathe, and R. B. Goldstein: "Environmental illness: a controlled study of 26 subjects with 20th century disease." *Journal of the American Medical Association,* 1990; 264:3166–3170.

Simon, G. E., W. J. Katon, and P. J. Sparks: "Allergic to life: psychologic factors in environmental illness." *American Journal of Psychiatry,* 1990; 147:901–906.

Terr, A. I.: "Clinical ecology in the workplace." *Journal of Occupational Medicine,* 1989; 31:257–261.

Terr, A. I.: "Environmental illness: a clinical review of 50 cases." *Archives of Internal Medicine,* 1986; 146:145–149.

METHODS

To review these articles I used the same criteria I use for any review of medical research. There are expected standards that medical science anticipates. My first question was, Is the article about multiple chemical sensitivity?

The authors of the *Journal of Occupational Medicine* article relied on the definition of MCS syndrome established by Dr. Mark Cullen ("Multiple chemical sensitivities: development of public policy in the face of scientific uncertainty." *New Solutions,* 1991; Fall: 16-24). Cullen's criteria are

1. MCS is **acquired** in relation to some documentable environmental exposure that may initially have produced a demonstrable toxic effect.

2. Symptoms involve **more than one organ system**, and recur and abate in response to **predictable** environmental stimuli.

3. Symptoms are elicited by exposures to chemicals that are **demonstrable** but very low.

4. **No** widely available **test** of organ system function can explain symptoms. (Quoted from the *Journal of Occupational Medicine* article, page 719.)

People have used numerous terms to describe the symptom set called MCS syndrome or other sets of symptoms that appear to be similar. Since

Dr. Cullen's definition is the one used by doctors practicing traditional medicine, as opposed to clinical ecology or environmental medicine, I looked for the authors' criteria to align with his.

The answer to my first question proved negative in every case, rendering further evaluation unproductive and unnecessary.

RESULTS

Paper One

Sparks, P. J., G. E. Simon, W. J. Katon, L. C. Altman, G. H. Ayars and R. L. Johnson: "An outbreak of illness among aerospace workers." *Western Journal of Medicine*, 1990; 153: 28–33.

Is the article about multiple chemical sensitivity? This paper discusses 53 subjects who filed for compensation following chemical poisoning. The background is given on page 28 of the paper:

> By mid–1988, more than half of the approximately 200 employees working with composite plastic materials in one building of a large aircraft manufacturing company reported multiple symptoms including dizziness, nausea, headaches, fatigue, shortness of breath, palpitations, and cognitive impairment. The composite materials were composed of fiberglass, graphite and other synthetic fibers. These fibers were impregnated with epoxies or phenol-formaldehyde resins and cured with heat to form rigid aircraft parts. For most workers, the symptoms were reported to begin within one week to six months after the introduction of fiberglass cloth impregnated with phenol-formaldehyde resin (phenolic material) in mid–1987 to comply with Federal Aviation Administration regulations regarding fire retardation.

Of the 200 workers reporting symptoms only 60 were selected for study. Seven of those workers failed to report for examination. That left a study group of 53. Study authors indicate that 15 of the subjects had symptoms consistent with multiple chemical sensitivity (MCS) syndrome, so 38 did not. Nevertheless all 53 subjects were studied.

Thus the nature of the study group poses two problems. First, what is the source of the conclusion that 15 of the subjects had symptoms consistent with multiple chemical sensitivity syndrome. It was not the study authors, for they did not provide diagnoses. The diagnoses were made by clinical physicians working for industry. The criteria by which the diagnoses were made is unknown. Second, data collection for the study failed to distinguish between patients with MCS symptoms and those without, as if the group of subjects were homogeneous. Homogeneity may have been based on the worksite, but not on the symptoms developed. Any special characteristics the MCS-symptomatic group may have had were lost to research.

Even laying aside the fact of an inappropriate study population, the authors' clear lack of understanding of MCS presents problems. For example, they note that "none of the workers tested had immunologin IgG or IgE antibodies to human serum albumin complexed with formaldehyde." It is ridiculous to imply that the lack of antibodies to formaldehyde indicates that these workers were not suffering disease from chemical exposure. It is true that certain individuals can develop specific respiratory sensitization to formaldehyde that results in an asthma-like picture, including the development of IgE and IgG antibodies. Antibodies have a half-life, however, and individuals who avoid contact with formaldehyde will eventually test negative for antibodies to it. Presence of antibodies is more likely a biomarker of toxic exposure than a measure of active disease. In general, testing MCS patients by focusing on antibodies to chemicals does not produce any significant findings.

One can only conclude that the study had nothing meaningful to say about multiple chemical sensitivity. The authors did not diagnose the subjects, nor did they include the criteria used for the second-hand diagnoses. Furthermore, the second-hand diagnoses of the 15 individuals was diluted by the use of 38 non–MCS symptomatic subjects. The best definition of the subjects is, perhaps, that they are one-quarter of a group of workers who reported adverse health effects from working with phenolic resins in aircraft manufacture. Using this study to conclude anything about individuals whose symptoms fit the criteria for multiple chemical sensitivity syndrome is impossible.

Paper Two

Simon, G. E., W. Daniell, H. Stockbridge, K. Claypoole, and L. Rosenstock: "Immunologic, psychological, neuropsychological factors in multiple chemical sensitivity." *Annals of Internal Medicine*, 1993; 119:97–103.

At first glance, this article certainly appears to address multiple chemical sensitivity. The study population allegedly had 41 subjects with chemical sensitivity and 34 control subjects. In this article as in the first one the authors did not diagnose multiple chemical sensitivity. The identification of those with MCS symptoms was made by Gordon P. Baker, M.D., a board-certified allergist. Of the 41 patients used in the study, only 18 had symptoms that fit the MCS profile according to Dr. Baker, which means that 23 did not. The 18 MCS patients were not a homogeneous group sharing a common toxic exposure. The authors do not identify the criteria used by Dr. Baker to identify MCS in the 18 patients. Nevertheless, all patients, MCS identified (18) and non–MCS identified (23), are grouped in the study as comprising a single group of 41 MCS subjects. The minute the two types of patients were grouped together, the paper ceased to be about multiple chemical sensitivity.

In the case of this particular paper there are some important issues to examine. Some journal articles exist in a virtual vacuum, but this paper and a number of others that have spun off the data have generated significant complaints. To understand part of the controversy, the reader must go back to September 12, 1991, when William Daniell, M.D., M.P.H., presented a paper called "A case-control comparison of immunologic and psychologic parameters in the multiple chemical sensitivity syndrome" to the Association of Occupational and Environmental Clinics. The study population and data for this paper are identical to that of Paper Two.

When papers share the same data, it would seem that information would be consistent. In this case the reverse occurs. The *Journal of Occupational Medicine* article refers to the study in Paper Two as "the one controlled and blinded" study in the literature on multiple chemical sensitivity (*Journal of Occupational Medicine*, 1994; 36(7), page 719). In his 1991 presentation of the same study, William Daniell made the statement that "all interviews were administered by one of the authors (G. E. [Simon]), who was not blind to case or control status." H. Stockbridge, another author, conducted neuropsychological interviews for the study, and he was not blinded either. Somehow, the research that was admittedly not blinded in 1991 had become blinded in later years.

When Paper Two was published Dr. Baker wrote a letter to *Annals of Internal Medicine* to clarify that only 18 of the 41 patients had been identified as having profiles consistent with MCSS. The journal chose not to print the letter, saying that it had arrived too late. The journal did, however, print six negative reviews of the article in February 1994.

Because of the problems inherent in this study, Albert Donnay, Executive Director of MCS Referral & Resources, Inc., filed a complaint with the Department of Health and Human Services Office of Research Integrity (ORI) on April 30, 1994. The issues were investigated at the direction of ORI. This type of investigation involves a review by appropriate officials in the institutions where the authors worked. The investigation was conducted primarily by the University of Washington with assistance from Group Health Cooperative. During the initial inquiry phase a comment addressed to "Associate Dean Dale Johnson, The Graduate School" June 6, 1994, from an unidentified person at the University of Washington (name blacked out) includes this statement:

> This paper is weak and should not have been published as it stands. Retraction of the paper should be considered as an option. *Publication of further papers on these data could destroy the reputations of the authors* [page 3 of the memo].

On the same page the author of the memo states, "This is just another weak paper put out by persons not familiar with a given methodology who have a previous bias."

The investigation, though it concluded nothing, led to the publication of a piece by R. A. Deyo, B. M. Psary, G. Simon, E. H. Wagner, and G. S. Omenn entitled "The messenger under attack — intimidation of researchers by special-interest groups." *New England Journal of Medicine*, 1997; 336:1176–1180. Three letters to the editor followed publication of this piece. Among the letters was the letter from Dr. Baker that *Annals of Internal Medicine* had failed to print. It read, in part:

> Believing the study planned to refine diagnostic criteria for multiple chemical sensitivity, I wanted to see how my assessments corresponded with the panel's conclusions.... [T]he researchers erroneously assumed that all 41 patients had multiple chemical sensitivity. In fact, a majority (23 of 41) did not, in my assessment as treating physician, fit the profile" [*New England Journal of Medicine*, 1997; 337:1314–1315].

In response to this letter in the same issue (pages 1315 to 1316), Drs. Simon and Deyo state:

> Dr. Baker consulted in designing the eligibility questionnaire, and his billing and chart diagnoses were used. Only after publication of the paper [Paper Two] did he question the diagnoses. He never responded to repeated requests to "rediagnose" the chemically sensitive group [page 1315].

A quick look back to the letters on the first publication, Paper Two, which appeared in Volume 20 of the 1994 issue of *Annals of Internal Medicine*, provides more detail on MCS subject selection:

Simon and colleagues selected patients with a computer billing code of multiple allergy, and then screened for illness lasting 3 months or more, multisystem involvement (including the central nervous system), and self-report of sensitivity to chemicals. With no screening for length, type or severity of exposure, level of sensitivity, or degree of illness, confounding variables remain unaddressed. Controls were not screened for sensitivity to chemicals, masked regular exposures, or previous occupations that could have provided chemical exposures [page 250].

Whether Dr. Baker's records were sufficient to identify multiple chemical sensitivity syndrome is doubtful. What is clear is that Dr. Baker identified only 18 of the 41 individuals as fitting the MCS symptom profile.

In their 1997 letter to the *New England Journal of Medicine* Drs. Simon and Deyo stated that "only after publication of the paper did he [Dr. Baker] question the diagnoses." This is not accurate unless the reference is to the premature "release of the unpublished study to the defense counsel in a major toxic-injury case, where it was used in cross-examination" (page 1315). That occurrence significantly predated publication and proved the cutoff in Dr. Baker's willingness to discuss any further issues on the data, including the number of patients he had identified as having profiles consistent with multiple chemical sensitivity syndrome symptoms. What is significant is that the authors went forward anyway, aware that the 41 lacked homogeneity.

Paper Two does not address multiple chemical sensitivity. Less than half the group fit the symptom profile. Just as in Paper One, any data that might have been gathered from MCS identified subjects in the group are diluted by the presence of non–MCS identified subjects, so the data are meaningless. It is perhaps noteworthy that readers of the 1993 Paper Two have no way to recognize its faults unless they also read the October 30, 1997, correspondence in the *New England of Medicine* about "The messenger under attack," published in the April 14, 1997, issue.

Paper Three

L. C. Grammer, K. E. Harris, M. A. Shaughnessy, P. Sparks, G. H. Ayars, and R. Patterson: "Clinical and immunologic evaluation of 37 workers exposed to gaseous formaldehyde." *Journal of Allergy and Clinical Immunology*, 1990; 86:177–181.

Is the article about multiple chemical sensitivity? The authors of this paper examine 37 patients who sought medical attention following airborne exposure to formaldehyde. There was no attempt to identify patient symptoms as fitting a profile for MCS. Furthermore, the authors again concentrated on immunologic factors, as we see from the following paragraph:

> The final evaluation for immunologically mediated disease was based on both the clinical and serologic assessments. None of the workers had IgE or IgG antibody to F [formaldehyde]-human serum albumin or an immunologic mediated respiratory or ocular disease caused by F; however, some of the workers appeared to experience irritant symptoms caused by workplace exposure to F or other irritant chemicals.

It is exceedingly unlikely that multiple chemical sensitivity is primarily related to immunologic factors. Lack of primary immunologic factors does not automatically rule out organic disease or disorder. The workers had exposure to phenol and methyl ethyl ketone, both of which can cause neurotoxic effects (which can be confused with psychogenic problems). The subjects in this study did not receive neurological testing, which might have produced significant findings.

This article should not be used as the basis for conclusions regarding MCS, because it isn't about multiple chemical sensitivity.

Paper Four

Black, D. W., A. Rathe, and R. B. Goldstein: "Environmental illness: a controlled study of 26 subjects with 20th century disease." *Journal of the American Medical Association*, 1990; 264:3166–3170.

The authors of this study focus on 26 subjects who had received a diagnosis of EI [environmental illness] from a clinical ecologist. The author explains EI this way: "The concept underlying EI is that common foods and chemicals create dysregulation of the immune system, which leads to the development of physical and mental disorders" [page 3166]. The authors made no attempt to link this study with multiple chemical sensitivity syndrome symptoms. This study has no place in the literature of MCS, because it isn't about multiple chemical sensitivity.

Paper Five

Simon, G. E., W. J. Katon, and P. J. Sparks: "Allergic to life: psychologic factors in environmental illness." *American Journal of Psychiatry*, 1990; 147:901–906.

This study uses 37 plastics workers for a study of psychological factors in environmental illness. The authors indicate that 13 subjects developed environmental illness. Using subjects with a condition termed environmental illness, the authors go on to conclude that "psychological vulnerability strongly influences chemical sensitivity following chemical exposure." The leap from environmental illness to chemical sensitivity is not justifiable. The article does not have anything to say about multiple chemical sensitivity.

Paper Six

Terr, A. I.: "Clinical ecology in the workplace." *Journal of Occupational Medicine*, 1989; 31:257–261.

Ninety cases were studied in which clinical ecologists made a diagnosis of environmental illness that resulted in a compensation claim. There was no use of research criteria for multiple chemical sensitivity, and the diagnosis of multiple chemical sensitivity was not made. The author did not provide the diagnoses. The article is not about multiple chemical sensitivity.

Paper Seven

Terr, A. I.: "Environmental illness: a clinical review of 50 cases." *Archives of Internal Medicine*, 1986; 146: 145–149.

This study consists of 50 cases. Patients were diagnosed with environmental illness by clinical ecologists. There was no use of research criteria, and the diagnosis of multiple chemical sensitivity was not made. This study is not about MCS.

DISCUSSION

In essence none of these seven articles written by prestigious researchers are about multiple chemical sensitivity, and serious charges of scientific misconduct have been leveled against the authors of one paper. Yet statements have been made, and policies developed, based on these papers with the assumption that they do apply to something called multiple chemical sensitivity. All of these seven studies are cited in the review articles by Sparks *et al.* to validate statements about multiple chemical sensitivity. Generally the theme of the review articles is to show that multiple chemical sensitivity has no immunologic component, has a high psychiatric component, has uncertain or no etiology, and needs to be treated and evaluated as a biopsychosocial disease by occupational medicine physicians, who have no training in this area. The absence of actual multiple chemical sensitivity patients in these studies is ignored.

How could such a distortion of the scientific method have occurred? Actually, the medical literature is full of similar distortions. For example, there was a report in 1922 of the successful treatment of schizophrenia, manic depressive illness, epilepsy, and a variety of psychotic conditions. The treatment was so good that only 42 of 1400 patients so treated returned to the hospital. It led to an increase in the discharge rate of 43 percent which produced some very happy physicians. The treatment: surgical removal of the colon. It was hailed as a medical miracle.

If perchance removal of the colon did not cure the patient ("cure" meant that the patient did not come back for further treatment), there were other things that could be removed: tonsils, teeth, cervix, uterus, gallbladder, appendix, ilium, or seminal vesicles. Those who subscribed to this theory believed that when the correct organ was removed the patient got better because the nidus of infection causing the psychosis or epilepsy was gone. Failure to respond meant that the wrong source of infection had been removed, so another one was chosen.

The predictable response of the patients were not to return to the hospital. It seems likely that they preferred continued illness to the prospect of more surgery. Chances are, their relatives agreed with them.

Could the authors of the review articles — purportedly articles about MCS — be similarly deluded? Perhaps. How, otherwise, could competent physician researchers convince themselves that they were studying one thing when they were actually studying another? Occupational medicine specialists insist that only they are qualified to diagnosis and treat people with multiple chemical sensitivity. This is despite the fact that they have no studies of the problem.

The conclusions the review authors reached on their non–MCS population so traumatized workers that they responded with anxiety, depression, and panic. This was a legitimate response to hearing that they had a disease that began with airborne chemical inhalation, had no etiology, was not related to the airborne chemical, and could strike at any time in an indiscriminate manner and leave them crippled for the rest of their lives. They were assured there was no known treatment and no known organic etiology. They learned that if they got the disease they would suddenly have developed a psychiatric condition that they could not understand, but they were assured that it would not be secondary to the airborne chemical exposure that started the problem.

As the researchers continued to study non–MCS patients and apply the findings to chemically poisoned patients, the chemically poisoned patients became increasingly emotionally alarmed, which strengthened the researchers' conviction that their theories about emotional illness were right. The patients reacted to this conviction with emotional responses of increasing severity, which eventually responded to the troublesome severity, which eventually added up to full-blown iatrogenic disease — that is, disease caused by the physician's treatment. Yet the possibility that patients' stress levels were rising as an effect of the lack of objectivity in research articles has been overlooked.

The vicious cycle goes on. As a result of their studies the researchers believe that chemical poisoning, the diagnoses of clinical ecologists, the scoring of three or more symptoms on a four-point scale, etc., represent multiple chemical sensitivity. Their studies of convenience, using others' diagnoses and having little or nothing in common with multiple chemical sensitivity, became models for research into multiple chemical sensitivity. As a result, chemical sensitivity is on the way to becoming a major national problem that did not have to be.

It is important to note that data may give the appearance of quality simply by being present in quantity. Placing these seven articles along with the two-part series from the *Journal of Occupational Medicine* out on a table might lead one to conclude that there has been some research on MCS. Let's summarize the number of subjects studied:

Papers	Number of subjects studied	Number of subjects with actual MCS symptoms
One	53	possibly 15
Two	41	18
Three	37	0
Four	26	0
Five	37	0
Six	90	0
Seven	50	0
Total	334	possibly 33

Though at first glance it appears that the combined articles offer research on 334 subjects with multiple chemical sensitivity, that is not the case. In fact, it would be safe scientifically to assume that none of the subjects were properly identified as having multiple chemical sensitivity, since not one author applies the label. (Furthermore, some of the studies may share subjects; 334 is the maximum possible number represented.)

Now, to apply the first question asked with respect to the claim that these articles have something to say about multiple chemical sensitivity: Papers Three through Seven do not identify populations as having symptoms characteristic of MCS. Paper One may have 15 subjects with symptoms consistent with MCS, but there is no way to determine the validity of that assumption. When all is said and done only 18 subjects from Paper Two can be said to have symptoms consistent with MCS, and those 18 were not diagnoses by the authors.

It is interesting to see articles written purporting to be providing useable information on multiple chemical sensitivity when in fact the authors never diagnose MCS. It is interesting to look at the display of these articles and realize that at most 33 individuals studied have the MCS symptom set. The only conclusion that can be drawn is that the seven papers have absolutely nothing to say about multiple chemical sensitivity.

For a two-part article entitled "Multiple Chemical Sensitivity Syndrome: A Clinical Perspective," one should expect that the authors would draw heavily on literature that involves research regarding MCS. This expectation is not met. Of the 98 references cited in the two articles only 17 titles even include the term "multiple chemical sensitivity."

It seems likely that anyone who studied a group of patients without MCS, then attempted to apply the generated data to another population of patients who do have MCS symptoms, might conclude the disease does not exist, since the data are not appropriate for the population. It is understandable that someone pursuing such a flawed line of study might come up with a statement such as Dr. Terr has made: "As defined and presented by its proponents, multiple chemical hypersensitivity constitutes a belief and not a disease" ("Multiple Chemical Sensitivities: Immunologic Critique of Clinical Ecology Theories and Practices," in *Occupational Medicine: State of the Art Reviews*, 1987; 2(4):693).* Of course, this line of study represents a belief system in itself: the belief that inappropriate data can successfully define the characteristics of a patient population. It is interesting

---

Information supplied by Albert Donnay, Executive Director, MCS Referral & Resources, Inc. 508 Westgate Road, Baltimore, Maryland 21229-2343, phone 410-362-6400.

that Dr. Terr feels qualified to make statements about MCS when he has stated that it is "out of his area" to "talk about toxic chemicals" (from a deposition taken in *Elizabeth Barbara Smith v. Oakland Hospital et al.*, before the California Workers' Compensation Appeals Board, April 24, 1985, p. 19).

It is possible that today's controversy arose out of the source of initial recognition of a problem. Doctors called clinical ecologists or environmental medicine doctors were among the first to identify the medical problem. At first the symptoms were thought to be related to allergy, so when Dr. Black in Paper Four addresses patient complaints of "candidiasis, immune dysregulation, cerebral allergy," it is little wonder that he was taken aback. Initial study of the problems did focus on the immune system. The immune system may be involved in the beginning by displaying some biomarkers of toxic exposure such as antibodies to various toxics, but in time those antibodies are gone, unless there is reexposure. Then they may reappear until the half life expires again. More is involved in disease than appearance of antibodies. Yet a debate on the immune system concerns many of the current authors even to the present. Those who are making progress in understanding this disease are pursuing study outside the field of immunology.

Multiple chemical sensitivity technically isn't a diagnosis. It is a syndrome, a group of symptoms that facilitates study. It is a temporary label for a symptom set, and for diagnostics to end there would be incomplete. One author has made a very salient point: Testing for the multiple chemical sensitivity patient should be individualized (Weaver, V. M., "Medical management of the multiple chemical sensitivity patient." *Regul Toxicol Pharmacol*, 1996; 24:1 Pt 2, S111-5). Individualized testing makes good common sense because one toxic may affect two individuals in two very different ways. Of course, these individual reactions present difficulties for researchers because all the cases do not fit neatly into one pattern.

As mentioned earlier, the authors of the *Journal of Occupational Medicine* two-part article draw on Dr. Mark Cullen's 1991 definition of multiple chemical sensitivity syndrome. At the same time, the authors note problems with this definition, including "the subjectivity and nonspecificity of information regarding 'predictable' and 'demonstrable' attributes of the exposure-symptom relationship." Actually, some of the difficulty in the literature comes not from those terms, but from the fourth part of Cullen's definition, which refers to the failure of available testing to adequately explain symptoms. The literature is filled with many articles essentially stating that since multiple chemical sensitivity is not an immune disease, it isn't a disease at all. Many of the papers reviewed here do just that; many of the authors were trying to disprove the existence of multiple chemical sensitivity as a disease because the immune profiles seemed to lack proof of disease. However, just because MCS isn't an immune disease does not mean it is not a disease or that it is not a constellation of diseases.

Dr. Cullen's definition includes an environmental exposure that produced a demonstrable toxic effect. Another term for demonstrable toxic effect is "toxic biomarker." There are numerous toxic biomarkers, including certain immune system antibodies.* A toxic biomarker is not an indicator of disease, but it is a clue to toxic exposure. Toxic exposures can poison. The appropriate place to start looking into an individual's potential MCS problem begins with poisoning. Has poisoning occurred? This is where the articles reviewed here spin off into strange territory.

On page 733 of the two-part *Journal of Occupational Medicine* article, a typical statement occurs: "Because there is *no* established and widely available test to use to diagnose MCS, the physician must be extremely cautious about excessive or inappropriate testing or the misinterpretation of these tests." They recommend only the following: 1. history, 2. physical examination, 3. consultation (occupational and environmental specialist, psychiatrist, other specialists as appropriate), 4. other (symptom diary, short-term removal from exposure) (page 733).

On page 734, the authors list a number of tests that they identify as not having been validated for confirming a diagnosis of multiple chemical sensitivity:

1. environmental challenge testing (uncontrolled, unblinded)
2. quantitative electroencephalography
3. brain electrical activity mapping
4. evoked potentials (brainstem, visual, sensory)
5. positron emission tomography scan
6. single photon emission computed tomography scan
7. immunologic testing
8. measurements of trace concentrations of volatile organic compound or pesticides in blood (parts per billion)
9. neuropsychologic testing

Multiple chemical sensitivity is a syndrome. It follows poisoning. *These tests were not designed for MCS, but they work remarkably well in identifying*

For in-depth information on effects-related biomarkers of toxic exposure the following website on the internet may be helpful: http://www.niehs.nih.gov/sbrp/newweb/resprog/pub/uwpub95.htm

damage resulting from poisoning. Individuals who have been identified as having MCS symptoms frequently will have positive results on these tests. Some results demonstrate severe levels of damage. Examples of results of poisoning shown by these tests are brain lesions, cognitive deficits, neurological damage and abnormal function, and vascular disease, to name a few. These results are typical of poisoning.

It is true there is no single, widely available test for MCS, but there are quite a number of tests for evidence of poisoning. These tests can also show what the results are not. For example, certain tests document profiles for obsessive compulsive disorder, Alzheimer's-type disease, and so on. The damage done by poisoning can be shown to be different from other established diseases and disorders.

On August 17, 1994, the Environmental Protection Agency published in the *Federal Register* its final report on "Principles of Neurotoxicity Risk Assessment." The following statement is found in the "Basic Neurotoxicological Principles" section 2.2.2:

> Neurotoxicity can be manifest as a structural or functional adverse response of the nervous system to a chemical, biological, or physical agent.... Neurotoxicity refers broadly to the adverse neural responses following exposure to chemical or physical agents (e.g., radiation). Adverse effects include any change that diminishes the ability to survive, reproduce, or adapt to the environment. Neuroactive substances may also impair health indirectly by altering behavior in such a way that safety is decreased in the performance of numerous activities.... The range of responses can vary from temporary responses following acute exposures to delayed responses following acute or chronic exposure to persistent responses. Neurotoxicity may or may not be reversible following cessation of exposures [page 42367].

In that publication (pages 42372 to 42378) there are a number of tests recommended to establish neurotoxicity. They include

> neurologic exam
> neuropsychological testing
> neurobehavioral tests
> computerized test batteries
> neurophysiologic tests (electromyographic responses, nerve conduction
>   velocity, electroencephalogram, evoked potentials)
> neurochemical tests
>   imaging techniques
>   thermography

> positron emission tomography
> magnetoencephalography
> magnetic resonance imaging
> spectroscopy
> computerized tomography
> doppler ultrasomography
> brain activity electrical mapping
> neuropathologic tests (biopsies of neurologic tissue)
> self-reporting methods
> mood scales
> personality scales

When this list is compared with the list of tests that the authors of the two-part *Journal of Occupational Medicine* reject, there is a striking similarity. The writing done by these authors focuses on the immune system and toxic exposure, not the nervous system; therefore they regard tests designed to examine the nervous system as useless. Certainly, one can, for example, agree that abnormal SPECT scan results don't directly diagnose MCS, but the results can be used to identify results of chemical poisoning.

The seven papers discussed in this chapter could simply be dismissed as poor science if they did not have such a significant effect on policy. That many of the articles are written by doctors who testify on behalf of various industries in toxic exposure cases is not, I think, coincidental. On page 718 of the *Journal of Occupational Medicine* article, this point is made right up front:

> There are significant ways in which the recognition of MCS as an occupational or environmental illness may interfere with the objective study of this phenomenon as a clinical condition. Recognition of this syndrome as an illness, with potential to cause permanent disability, could involve changes in health care coverage and delivery, awarding of workers' compensation benefits, and the regulation of chemicals in the workplace and the environment in the United States.

In the second part, the article discusses history taking, physical exam, consultation, and other workups. That many physicians would have difficulty with the recommendation for evaluation should not be surprising. For example, the authors suggest that "any technique for investigating the central nervous system effects of low-level exposure to chemical substances should only take place in a research setting with proper controls to validate its clinical use as a diagnostic tool to confirm the presence of MCS" (page 733). This sounds quite logical until one leaves the world of the theoretical and enters reality.

The places where research of this nature might occur are frequently funded by sources that have an intense interest in the outcome of the MCS debate. For those researchers or treating physicians who gain insight into the MCS condition, the disincentives to proceed are often overwhelming. Nevertheless, information with respect to low-level poisoning and its results in the human is accumulating daily. Part of the reason for the growth of knowledge is the view that if poisoning has occurred, the search for results of that poisoning should begin. The tools for that search are already available and in use.

The authors of the two-part article may not be aware of the use of these tests because they are from disciplines that do not routinely use them. Of the seven authors, the following fields are represented: occupational medicine, psychiatry, allergy, and immunology. The absence of a voice from the field of neurology may account for the manner in which they view MCS and dismiss tests which show abnormalities in the MCS identified group.

The second part of the article also contains a section on treatment. In this area the recommendations could be described as utterly irresponsible. The article states (page 732):

The fact that there is no agreement upon any one etiology for most patients with MCS does not prevent clinicians from helping affected patients with their symptoms. [Italics in original.]

To leap to treatment without knowledge of what the problem is can be hazardous to the health of the patient. Examples of treatment suggestions from pages 734 to 735 follow

> The goal of therapy is control of symptoms, and success is not dependent upon a specific organic diagnosis or etiology but rather on the patient's improved understanding of the role of stress on his or her illness and the acquisition of skills for coping with the impact of the illness on daily life.

> A multidisciplinary and behavioral medicine approach similar to that taken in the treatment of pain, which also may or may not have objective physical correlates, may help the patient cope better with his or her symptoms.

> Psychiatric treatments may be helpful in controlling symptoms *regardless* of etiology.

> Pharmacologic treatment may be a helpful adjunct....

> A definite medical recommendation for complete avoidance of chemical exposure is not indicated at this time.

[127]

First, the authors admit they do not know the etiology or the processes of MCS. They assume that MCS is psychogenic, and their recommendations proceed from that assumption.

From reading the articles, it is not clear whether any of the authors have ever seen a patient with MCS. It is clear that they have not diagnosed one. I have seen some MCS patients, as well as a patient diagnosed by another doctor as suffering environmental illness. The one with the diagnosis of environmental illness did not have symptoms like the ones with the MCS symptom set. On the tests I ran, the environmental illness patient had normal test values. The MCS patients, in contrast, often demonstrated an array of bizarre abnormalities. Duplicate individual tests validated the results.

Aside from brain abnormalities consistent with toxic effects found in those poisoned by petroleum products, corrosive aromatics, acids, caustic alkalis, nonpetroleum solvents, carbon monoxide, and other fumes or gases, some of these patients have developed toxic-induced porphyrias, asthma or asthma-type respiratory difficulty, and vascular disease. The patients had a number of other medical conditions tied directly to poisoning. To make the statement that avoidance of chemical exposure is not indicated is irresponsible. Patients have become financially bankrupt, had their health deteriorate at quicker rates than necessary, lost supportive friends and family because of such irresponsible writing and readers who have little experience evaluating medical writing. In trying to follow recommendations for treatment as given by the authors, some patients have been seriously harmed.

Even worse, this literature is establishing a national database upon which health care policy decisions are being made. The United States is producing federal MCS policy based upon a database that has nothing whatever to do with MCS. Taxpayer dollars are going into development of a monumental problem where policy is being developed and will be applied to the chemically injured despite the fact that the policy has nothing to do with their illness. Time, effort, and money is being spent on something that is worse than nothing. This effort hinders real progress and requires more time to correct. In addition, these policy decisions may be made in an atmosphere of fear instead of reason. The idea of the enormity of the MCS problem based on the popular figure of 15 percent of the population's having chemical sensitivity is not indicative of MCS in its disabling form. Yet fears of the costs of recognition of 37 or more millions of people with disabling MCS seems to cause both governmental inaction due to erroneous perceptions of economic disaster and active creation of a profusion of unscientific literature that create confusion instead of contributing fact. Demands are made such as requiring controlled, double-blind studies before recognizing this medical condition, as if any other studies would be unscientific. Multiple sclerosis (MS), for example, has no known etiology. Lack of controlled, double-blind studies does not prevent real scientists from performing real scientific studies with respect to MS or doctors from diagnosing the disease. We would never have been able to put a rocket — let alone man — on the moon if controlled double-blind studies were required in science.

Many chemical sensitives can and do work. Doctors who accept and treat these patients recognize the problem. It's a problem of chemical poisoning. They know the tests to use and they apply them. They do not get caught in repetitive traps: "MCS is not an immune problem and therefore not a disease" or "there is no specific test for MCS therefore MCS is not a disease" and "there is no evidence at this time that avoidance of chemical exposure is recommended" as if by repeating non-science it would become science by virtue of repetition. Science probes to *answer* questions and, once answered, there is always the realization that the results may be wrong. Dogmatic insistence that a series of tests be ignored made by those who do not use those tests is unscientific arrogance. Until the pursuit becomes one of the scientific probing to determine the results of chemical poisoning in an individual experiencing effects of toxic exposure we will ultimately base national policy on non-science and medical science will lose credibility.

Objective studies of chemical poisoning and sensitivity go back a long way. In 1966 the Medical Annals of the District of Columbia published research by E. W. Kailin concerning the effects of DDT on human subjects. (Kailin, E. W., "Electromyographic evidence of DDT-induced myasthenia." *Medical Annals of the District of Columbia*, 1966; 35:237–245. Kailin, E. W., "Cerebral disturbances from small amounts of DDT." *Medical Annals of the District of Columbia*; 1966; 35:519–524.) Dr. Kailin measured the electromyographic effects of exposure to minute amounts of DTT under controlled conditions. She exposed sensitive and nonsensitive human subjects to infranasal concentrations of 10 ppm, 100 ppm, and 1000 ppm. These doses markedly inhibited the amplitude of the electromyographic potentials within minutes. Her evidence indicated that the site of the DDT action was in the central nervous system and not at the myoneural junction (the point at which the nerve stimulates the muscle). Thus this doctor, more than 30 years ago, developed a method of studying sensitivity (or poisoning) by odors with a simple, objective test. Her research was never followed up.

SUMMARY

This chapter has attempted to bring to the reader's attention the following facts:

1. There are no studies on multiple chemical sensitivity on which to base informed policy decisions.

2. The collection and interpretation of data is subject to distortions and delusions that sometimes make reasonable policy or studies impossible.

3. Multiple chemical sensitivity has none of the characteristics of an immunologic disease, and as long as immunologic criteria are required as proof of its existence, it will be seen as a non-disease.

4. Objective data for the study of MCS were developed in 1966 and, if used, would have avoided the present fanatical arguments pro and con and saved enormous amounts of money and energy in researching chemical sensitivity.

Furthermore, doctors need not seek a test specifically for MCS. They can and do recognize the root cause as toxic, and they can examine and evaluate signs of poisoning. The varied symptoms are real diseases, including asthma, toxic encephalopathy, vascular disease, peripheral neuropathy, and porphyria. It could be said that MCS is a convenient framework that permits examination of a type of poisoning.

Recommended Reading

The following two articles provide additional information on issues explored in this chapter:

Davidoff, A. L., and L. Fogarty: "Psychogenic origins of multiple chemical sensitivities syndrome: a critical review of the research literature." *Archives of Environmental Health*, 1994; 49(5):316–325.
Davidoff, L. L.: "Models of multiple chemical sensitivities (MCS) syndrome: Using empirical data (especially interview data) to focus investigations." *Toxicology and Industrial Health*, 1992; 8(4):229–247.

PERSONAL EXPERIENCE
WITH MCS

Look at me. Unless I'm in an obvious state of intoxication from some neurotoxic or porphyrinogenic substance, I look just like any normal human. You'd never guess what my brain is doing to generate that normal look. You don't know that I see multiples of you; that despite my effort, after we talk I can remember little of what was discussed; that when I shift my eyes from one place to another, or move my arm, I feel a shock like you might if you walked across a carpet and grabbed a doorknob. Nor can you hear the ringing in my ears that never goes away. Unless something is apparent on the surface, you will miss it. That's why it's time for me to share my experience — so that others can get some idea of what the chemical assault it.

I agreed to write about my experience with chemical sensitivity before I really thought about the manner in which it should be done, how difficult it would be to accomplish, and what effect it might have on me. I know that I serve as a virtual storehouse of experience — mine and that of other chemically injured workers in my own state (Washington) and elsewhere. To put that information together in a smooth, coherent, easily readable manner might have been possible, before I was poisoned. But the skills I once had have been severely compromised.

To begin this effort I gathered together my medical record, my "Timeline of Problems with the Office of Workers' Compensation Programs (OWCP)," and the "Annotated Timeline for MCS Related Events in Washington State," a document assembled December 14, 1994, by Faye Schrum, a support group leader for chemically injured Boeing workers; Kate Austin, advocate for injured workers in Washington State; and me.

As I began to piece together my experience using these documents as guides, I struggled with the question of how much detail to include. In recent years people in the United States have become accustomed to a diet of sound bites, not a full meal of in-depth information that requires significant thought and reasoning. At the same time, the public discounts the validity of sound-bite information because supporting data are missing.

It seemed to me that if I put together a piece that glossed over my experience and required little thought, more people might read it, but the validity of the material would be discounted. Furthermore, I'd be missing an opportunity to make several significant points whose veracity is documented by my experience:

- That chemical sensitivity is a major health problem, not a psychogenic creation in the minds of people who don't wish to work.
- That its prevalence increases exponentially while it is carefully ignored by those who could stop it.
- That doctors and officials (including workers compensation officials) have knowingly covered up the problem by corrupting the very systems that should protect the public.
- That the checks and balances of government at the state and federal levels are caught in deep rust (scales of justice rusted tight cannot weigh anything.)
- That although the medical problem is real, the notion of justice for the chemically sensitive is a figment of the imagination.

Millions of chemically injured people nationwide have run headlong into the same problems I face. Recently the news has focused on the health problems of Gulf War vets. Their problems are similar to those of the chemically injured. They know it. But the people with black lung disease working in the coal mines have been where we are; the Vietnam vets with Agent Orange exposure have been where we are. It's nothing new. One of my concerns is that society is so entrenched in its learned behavior with respect to the way these cases are handled that it seems incapable of changing.

It's much more fun for the public to watch a soft news program pit business and industry "experts" against the chemically injured than to listen attentively to real investigative reporting. Besides, there isn't much of the latter. Entertainment, however, soon loses its value when the problem hits home.

What I've decided to do with this section is to take the reader with me as I describe and document my experience. The chance of losing readers who find it boring is one I'm willing to risk for the gain of those who do stay with it and understand or at least ask themselves, "What if this is true?" I am also willing to risk the likelihood that some who do read it will respond with assurance that I am crazy.

For those willing to dig, following the action of OWCP officials over time will provide a picture of atrocities that the United States taxpayer has supported without knowledge. The integrity of the medical system in the United States will present itself in a way for which many will be unprepared. This section will show some problems that need to be solved. They will never be solved until the public knows they exist and insists that something be done.

The section begins by describing how I was first injured. That injury resulted immediately in moderate brain impairment, disorder of porphyrin metabolism in four of five tested areas, and asthma. Along with countless others I fell into a labeling system that was medically expeditious. The constellation of our symptoms came to be called multiple chemical sensitivity syndrome (MCSS), or chemical sensitivity. The fact that chemical sensitivity didn't jump right out of medical reference books did not make it nonexistent or, as some have suggested, a fabrication to which people turn when they reject a psychiatric diagnosis of their problems.

Technically I am a victim, though I haven't yet learned the right behavior for victims. As this experience unfolds chronologically, a healthy reader with some effort can accompany me. To accompany me without personal chemical injury makes it difficult to share the experience fully, but that may not be necessary. Follow a thread: Watch what the U.S. taxpayer pays OWCP officials to do; watch what doctors do for OWCP; watch how economic pressure influences political agendas.

Above all else, *watch*.

I couldn't breathe properly. I chalked it up to allergy, and I took an antihistamine. The antihistamine did nothing. I felt as if I were covered in the perfume, thick as honey, and I couldn't get it off. I left the area briefly. Cleaner air seemed to help, but my head hurt, and I wondered why I couldn't breathe. Under the circumstances, I decided to do what most workers might do in such an odd situation: I denied there was a problem and returned to my office. I sat down at the computer to begin my work. The computer looked like something I'd never seen before. I didn't have any idea what to do with it. I began to realize there was a real problem here.

I remember only a few other things that happened that day. I recall that out in the halls I could identify where every person had been. They left trails of scent — perfume, hairspray, lack of personal hygiene, and other odors. Each was distinct, and all were equally discernible simultaneously. I could have followed any one of them blindfolded. I did not want that knowledge.

From that day I lost the concept of what normal is. My ears were constantly ringing. I couldn't get thoughts to line up right. Even with the crutches I often felt as if I were about to fall. There was nausea. Occasionally I experienced what I came to call my brain turning off. It's as if I were missing for brief periods. From time to time I'd miss chunks of what people were saying to me. Occasionally my utterances became garbled; a syllable from one word would attach to another, or words would transpose, or a simple word just ran off and hid. Other times I'd try to tell someone something and completely lose track of what I was saying. Trying to reconstruct the conversation didn't help a bit. And then, there was this short-circuiting of my electrical system. I didn't know what else to call it. If I moved my eyes, I felt shock in my eyes. If I turned my head I felt shock. If I moved an arm, the shock was there. While all this was occurring, I tried to act as normal as possible and do my work despite the fact that my vision was creating problems. I managed, until pain hit my right side and then my left side. The pain was so severe it would bring me to my knees.

From October 1988 to January 1989 I spent as much time at work as I could stand. When that was too difficult, I went downtown to a respiratory specialist's office. He did standard tests and tried to treat my breathing problem. He informed me right away that the perfume probably set the problem off but was unlikely as the cause. He gave me Medrol, a steroid, to reduce inflammation. I had a systemic reaction to the drug. He gave me an antibiotic, since x-rays showed pneumonia. I had a systemic reaction to the antibiotic. He gave me inhalers to use for asthma, a condition I'd never had. I was to report to him any time I found the workplace causing me problems. My supervisor's entries in my workers' compensation file show that between October 24, 1988, and January 20, 1989, I required 72 hours of leave due to the condition.

At first the inhalers helped, but something at work was literally driving me wild. Weekends seemed to help me recover, but the reintroduction to work was a disaster — no matter how I tried to deny there was a problem.

There came a time when I found the inhalers were not helping. The doctor increased the dosage. The more he increased it, the less able I was to tolerate it. At that point I was fighting to continue working. I began losing weight. I was exhausted. One day I told the doctor the inhalers were not making me better but were contributing to the problem. They opened me up briefly, I explained, and then they shut me right back down. I explained that I'd rather just deal with the initial bronchoconstriction and not add the effect of the inhalers on top of that.

A pulmonologist worth his salt just can't deal with comments like that. Normal asthmatics can handle inhalers. From that moment, my doctor's perception of my condition had to change. I am not a normal asthmatic. My respiratory problem isn't standard asthma exactly. Of course, pulmonologists don't even agree on the definition of asthma, but when inhalers contribute to the problem, something is abnormal.

This doctor did not give up easily. He kept on trying. He researched, but found no satisfactory answers. His standard removal and return-to-work trials made the location of the source clear: It was something at work. But what, exactly? The doctor decided to send me to an allergist/immunologist.

It took some time to get an opening with the doctor to whom I was referred. I told him what had been happening. He did a few allergy tests, but they showed little and gave no definitive answer. After he ran some other tests through a lab in California, I returned to his office to see what he'd learned. I remember that he spoke gently. "Bonnye, you've been poisoned. Until the workplace is cleaned up, you cannot go back there." I can remember sitting there and seeing that he was talking, but I felt as if I were a million miles away. The word "poisoned" had never entered my mind. I thought of the Borgias and macabre things. I thought of bottles with the skull and crossbones. I thought of Mr. Yuck. How had a simple "allergy" changed into something like poisoning?

[137]

Following the meeting with the allergist/immunologist, I went to work January 20, 1989, and talked with people in the personnel office. I told them a doctor had advised me not to work in that office until the problem was fixed. Ironically, at that point I had no doubt that either the workplace would eventually become tolerable or whatever problem I was experiencing would pass. I really had no concept that I might be disabled to any extent that would prohibit me from working in the future, but I did recognize that I had to find some way for my body to deal with routine chemicals which were intoxicating me. Personnel office officials suggested I file for disability retirement as well as workers' compensation. I took the forms and began the process. They placed me on an indefinite leave without pay status.

The supervisor's report on the accuracy of the records I sent in my workers' compensation claim reads: "On 24 October 1988 Bonnye appeared to have a serious allergic reaction — she had difficulty breathing, her face appeared 'flushed' and she was not thinking clearly.... She continued to have discomfort after the initial allergic reaction." This report admitted that most of the chemicals I documented as toxic air contaminants in the building were in fact present. In this case I was very fortunate. Most individuals made sick by indoor air find that their employer will not support them.

The allergist/immunologist's test data identified an allergic immunoglobulin response to trimellitic anhydride (TMA). I called Northwest Environmental Services, Inc., out of the phone book and talked to their director of air studies. I asked about the chemical and explained my problem. The director asked where I got sick. I told her at work. She said that the source of TMA must be at work, then. I asked her where in a workplace office environment she'd look for TMA. Her immediate response was, "The carpet."

I asked for a sample of the carpet at work but was never permitted to have one. I asked the contracting department to get me the list of materials the contractor had used when the carpet was laid in the spring of 1987. The contracting department responded that the contractor's records had burned and were no longer available.

I tried to get my employer to let me work at home. The answer was negative. For medical reasons I had to leave my job — a job that I loved. I filed for workers' comp and for disability retirement. Completing forms covering all the information was a time-consuming process. Once the papers were filed, I had to deal with different thoughts. I asked the question everyone asks: "Why me?" Then I moved on to a more important question. *What next?*

I have lots of skills. There have been titles: English teacher, French teacher, proofreader, trainer, commercial casualty underwriter, employee development specialist, personnel management specialist, principal classifier, chief of classification and performance management. Always when I moved from job to job what people remembered was that I focused on solving problems. Now I was surrounded by problems to solve. I knew I had to learn about this thing, provide information to others, and do what I could to save others from this fate.

I asked the personnel officer to request an air study in my office building. They had done many in that building, since complaints were frequent. At length the air study was complete, with these findings:

22 Employees in Personnel Office

10 employees with no adverse health effects	*12 employees with adverse health effects*
5 complained about temperature	8 had adverse health effects
5 had no complaints at all	4 had two or more adverse health effects
(group contained 4 smokers)	(group contained 1 smoker)

I asked for the air study to determine whether they could find TMA. Also, I asked if they could identify a white powder that had frequently fallen from the ceiling onto my clothing while I worked. The industrial hygienist who did the air study in 1989 for the Department of Health and Human Services, Public Health Service, indicated he could find no TMA. The carpet, however, was laid in 1987, and another industrial hygienist explained that instruments were not calibrated to identify the low levels of TMA that would remain after that period of time. In other words, the air study could state that no TMA was found, but it could not certify that none was present. Equipment was not designed to test for zero. As for the white powder, the only response I ever got to my repeated queries was that it wasn't asbestos.

I remembered the carpet installation. I remembered the feel of the wet carpet on my feet when I would slip my shoes off under my desk. I remembered the odor. I remembered, too, that the contractor came back later to put the baseboard in place — another use of TMA.

Meanwhile I returned to the pulmonologist who had referred me to the allergist-immunologist. He decided to send me to another doctor and said he'd let me know when the appointment was set. After leaving his office on one of these visits, I remember driving around the downtown area. Suddenly it struck me that I was supposed to be headed for home. I have no idea what caused me to drive aimlessly through unfamiliar areas, or how long I had been doing it before I became aware that I was wandering. I do know that a great horror overcame me. It was one of my first serious encounters with severe "brain fog." Later when I'd find that somehow I'd overshot a destination by several blocks (or miles) it didn't come as such a shock. The first time, it can be a shattering experience and can easily cause the victim to question his own sanity.

About that time, my workplace was required to enter into Reduction-in-Force (RIF), and I received a RIF notice. I was told that I would be entitled to severance pay and unemployment compensation. At that time I received neither. Unemployment compensation was out of the question, because to qualify I would have to be actively seeking work. I didn't fully understand what was wrong with me, but I knew that at least for the time being, job hunting was impossible. When I drove in traffic, the vehicle exhaust made me sick. Perfume made me sick. I had asked my employer if I could work at home, and I had been turned down. Where could I go? The answer seemed to be "nowhere."

I began to study, reading everything I could dig up. Other people with similar problems began to contact me, and eventually we held two well-attended public meetings.

At these meetings it became clear that many attendees were having difficulty with the state workers' compensation program, called L & I (short for Labor and Industries). I knew that these injured workers needed a law somewhere at the state level that recognized their chemical sensitivity. It occurred to me that persuading the state to grant disabled parking permits to chemical sensitives would be a good approach. It would provide the necessary "ink on paper," and I knew from experience that chemically injured people needed disabled parking. I had once walked into my family doctor's office after passing a parked car that was leaking something awful. On entering the doctor's office, I promptly walked into a wall. (The doctor sent me for an MRI looking for an acoustical neuroma.)

I contacted my representatives in the state legislature. They asked me to get letters from all over the state, if possible, to indicate there was a problem. That was not difficult. The leaders of the informational meetings (myself included) drafted a letter and sent a copy to the people who had attended the meetings. We asked them to write the legislators if they felt the disabled parking was important. We also suggested that they have others who recognized the need to do the same thing. The response was tremendous. And the wheels began to turn.

While I was involved in all this activity, the workers' compensation officials on my case had sent my initially filed papers to a doctor for review. I had no knowledge of the action. The doctor, who never saw me or talked to me, diagnosed "aggravation of a mucosal irritation."

Meanwhile, it had taken only two weeks for the Office of Personnel Management to accept my claim for disability retirement. I was holding off on initiating the payments, however, because of some misinformation I had been given, which had led me to believe that accepting disability payments would disqualify me from receiving workers' compensation. I felt that workers' comp was the appropriate relief for my financial problems, since the injury happened at my workplace. So I continued to pursue that avenue.

In the hope of accelerating the action on my workers' compensation claim, I decided to find an attorney. The search was long and difficult. I could not find anyone in Seattle willing to handle a federal workers' comp case. At last I was given the name of an attorney in Tacoma.

When I first arrived at the office of the attorney, Matthew Sweeting, his first question was whether I'd seen a clinical psychologist who was testing for organic brain syndrome. After the drive to Tacoma in the polluted air of the freeway, I had enough difficulty walking that the attorney was able to see it. I was unfamiliar with the term "organic brain syndrome" despite my contact with others who had been poisoned. I told Mr. Sweeting that the allergist/immunologist had asked whether I had any difficulty thinking, but I didn't believe I did. Mr. Sweeting urged me to see the clinical psychologist anyway, and I assured him I'd go.

I asked why so few attorneys seemed willing to take a case involving federal workers' compensation. He told me that it was a matter of money. In the state system attorneys could go contingency, but the federal system tells attorneys what they can charge and for what. Few attorneys find it economically feasible to take these cases, which involve a great deal of labor in dealing with the convoluted Federal Employees Compensation Act and with sometimes difficult employees at the Office of Workers' Compensation Programs. Nevertheless, at the end of our meeting, Matt Sweeting agreed to represent me.

IV : Personal Experience with MCS

On May 5, 1989 I attended a program called "Recent Developments in Occupational Medicine — MCSS" at the Northwest Center for Occupational Health and Safety at the University of Washington. One of the main presentations was a paper called "Psychiatric Perspectives on MCSS." The author's view about chemical sensitivity syndrome, which he taught at the University of Washington as well as at this meeting, was that

> certain psychological vulnerabilities strongly influence the development of MCSS following an environmental insult or exposure. Possible mechanisms for this influence include behavioral conditioning, "masked" psychiatric illness, and somatization/hypochondriasis. All mechanisms may contribute, and each has important implications for treating symptoms and reducing disability.

The meeting was long, and though one participant did seem to suggest there were no real data to prove that the condition was largely psychologic, the prevailing sentiment was clearly in favor of the paper just quoted. I was amazed that the doctor who wrote that paper had the temerity to speak with so much certainty on a subject that obviously he did not understand.

I went to the clinical psychologist my attorney suggested. She saw me at a doctor's office in the city of Auburn, where people with MCS symptoms seemed to do better than in Seattle. I went in with no idea what was coming next. We talked for a time, and then the neuropsychological testing began. It was simple stuff, really — for a short time.

My first hint of what organic brain syndrome involved — my first realization of what it had done to me — came when the clinical psychologist asked me to do a simple math problem. Now, math was my forte. I always scored very high on math tests. In college, I had majored in English Education because I wanted to be well rounded.

I knew the math process, of course. But as soon as I began calculating, the numbers disappeared from my mind. I couldn't believe what was happening. I sat there baffled. I asked, "Would you repeat that?" The psychologist did. The same thing happened. I looked at her.

"This is where I feel like that wicked witch of the west," she said.

I knew that something had happened to my brain. My mind's eye was blind. I was devastated and fascinated at the same time. How could this have happened without my knowing it? As we went on, I saw more areas of dysfunction. When the testing was complete, the results showed that I did have organic brain syndrome, and my IQ was labeled at 115. I wasn't sure what that meant, but one thing seemed clear: I could no longer perform in ways I had counted on in the past.

Shortly thereafter I received a call from my supervisor, who was relaying a question for one of the colonels at work. If all the carpet was pulled out of the building and replaced, would I be able to return to the office?

I was deeply touched by the offer, and terribly torn. I had just become acutely aware that I had experienced brain damage. Significant parts of my brain were no longer functioning normally. I knew that glued-down carpet such as they used at my office was attached with the type of glue that had poisoned me once already (despite the label it carries of "no known health hazards"). The colonel had no idea that his suggestion was that I experience again what I had just experienced. Yet, I wanted desperately to return to work. I had taken a downgrade to work at the Corps. I was in a GS-11 level job; qualified for non-competitive employment at GS-12; and listed as "exceptional" for the army's career program for GM-13 personnel officer. My personnel officer was soon to retire. I wanted to compete for that job.

I considered with no little gratitude the offer. The building is one of the largest floor-surface area office buildings in the Seattle metropolitan area. It would be expensive to do what the colonel offered. At the same time I had my own view of the amount of TMA off-gassing in that area, both from new carpet and carpet glue. In a matter of seconds I had to overcome denial that at least for a time, my career had in fact died, taking opportunity along with it. My grief increased. I was too sick to accept the offer.

While all this was going on, I was stunned to receive a notice that my health insurance had passed the conversion date. I had never given a thought to losing my insurance, since it was available through disability retirement. But I was still holding on initiating that program. I contacted the people who sent me the letter and asked whether I might have a conversion deadline waiver due to my having organic brain syndrome.

I was granted the waiver, and I did have a conversion policy for a brief period of time, though the rate was exorbitant. The insurer made it very clear that with organic brain syndrome I was uninsurable. Had I not qualified by right of conversion, I could not have obtained insurance. That was another blow. My brain. My career. Insurability. (Later, I discovered that I had actually had insurance all the time, but I could not recover the unnecessary payment for the conversion policy.)

Following my testing with the clinical psychologist, I saw a psychiatrist, who concurred with the diagnosis of organic brain syndrome. I can remember sitting in his office occasionally after significant exposure. Sometimes he'd ask what was going on in my mind. There were times I'd have to answer honestly, "Nothing." That was another horrifying aspect of organic brain syndrome that revealed itself. I could not have imagined such a thing prior to poisoning. I know now what it is to experience days in which not a single thought passes in my brain. My mind registers events as they occur, but the constant flow of thoughts that used to mark my waking hours sometimes disappeared altogether. I might as well have been a tree.

I also remember the psychiatrist doing something I had never seen a doctor do. One day, I was describing the need for energy when I felt so tired. I told him I had discovered how to get that energy: I could go to a service station and pump gas. It made me sick, but it gave me a burst of odd, hyperactive energy. The psychiatrist exploded, frightening me out of my wits. He told me that what I said made as much sense as reaching into my head, grabbing a handful of brain cells, and beating them to death with a hammer. Contact with gasoline was killing brain cells. His dramatic manner certainly impressed me. After that, I was much more careful about what I exposed myself to.

Finally the pulmonologist called with his referral. The doctor he'd wanted me to see was out of town, so he scheduled me with two other doctors, both in the occupational medicine program at Harborview Hospital, an affiliate of the University of Washington.

At the same time my workers' comp officials informed me that I was scheduled to see yet another doctor at the same office. When they learned that I already had an appointment at that clinic, they decided my already scheduled appointment would suffice for their purposes.

I kept that appointment in May 1989. The doctors were very informal. They assured me that I probably knew more about multiple chemical sensitivity syndrome than they did. I did not agree or disagree; I only wondered, if that were true, why I was there. They knew about my activities and that I was planning to write a book.

Though the meeting seemed superficial, I did have some upsetting experiences. First of all, I was dismayed to discover how much weight I had lost. Since October 1988 I had steadily lost weight, even though I con-sumed about 5000 calories a day hoping to maintain. From October 1988 to May 1989 I had lost 22 pounds. I also was disturbed by a breathing test. I had had no difficulty breathing that day, but as soon as the technician entered the room, problems began. She was wearing scented lip gloss. The initial test set the base, and the second test, after use of an inhaler, showed increased bronchoconstriction. That confirmed what I'd been saying about inhalers, but it baffled the doctors.

These doctors sent me to a psychiatrist, apparently at the request of workers' comp officials. Their choice was a doctor at the Center for Anxiety and Depression at the University of Washington.

The psychiatrist's appointment was difficult for me. He had certain personal habits that I found embarrassing and distracting, greatly adding to my difficulty in concentrating. The main thing I remember is that he asked me to subtract a two-digit number from a two-digit number in my head. When I couldn't do it, he wrote the problem on paper, held it up for me, and asked me to try again. It took a little time, but I was able to do it. He congratulated the clinical psychologist for her success in identi-fying such a subtle thing as this organic brain syndrome.

The psychiatrist's report was a disturbing surprise and made me angry. Ignoring the symptoms of organic brain syndrome that he himself had noted, he speculated that I might have possible "masked" psychiatric prob-lems. He tried, however, to have it both ways, going on to say:

> ...a psychiatric or psychological explanation would never be acceptable to her. It is for this reason that the patient was told that she had no definite, treatable, major psychiatric disorder which is in a sense true.

The rest of his report is characterized by the same sort of waffling, but he makes several clear statements. He cautioned against a trial of psychi-atric drugs, noting that not only would they be unlikely to improve my symptoms, but they might produce a hypersensitivity reaction. "More importantly," he goes on, "I believe that indeed the patient is one of a num-ber of people who have clear-cut increase in sensitivity to various toxins."

Overall, I found the psychiatrist's report contradictory and confusing, but it was not up to me to interpret it. That was the job of the Harborview doctors who referred me to interpret this report, and they informed OWCP that the doctor had not identified any psychiatric problems. The result was good news: Based on the three doctors' reports, OWCP accepted that I was suffering from "work-related aggravation of mucosal irritation and multiple chemical sensitivity syndrome." Since organic brain syndrome is part of the MCS syndrome and since the clinical psychologist and two psychiatrists (theirs and mine) had recognized it, that was part of the MCS condition that OWCP accepted. Based on this acceptance, I was to begin receiving compensation as well as reimbursement for medical expenses.

My hope had finally found substance. I was elated. Now, I thought, I can really get to the bottom of what is making me sick. I saw the psychiatrist I had chosen on my own briefly to help me deal with the anger that the medical report engendered and the fact that the other psychiatrist had lied to me.

In July of 1989 the Boeing Company published a document, "IME Protocol for Chemical Claims" (author unidentified). Though I was unaware of the document at the time (I first saw it in 1996), I mention it here because the significance of this publication (and its date) cannot be overstated. In this document, Boeing lays out exactly what tests should be run on chemically injured claimants in order to substantiate their claims. These data were so well informed that it took the rest of the country three to four years to catch up. IME doctors I saw had already seen this document.

An IME is an independent medical exam, something often required to complete a workers' comp claim. Included in Boeing's instructions to IME doctors is the following information:

> Effects of solvent exposure on the central nervous system (CNS) may be manifested as a mental disorder, an impairment in psychologic functioning, or as nerve damage. Symptoms resulting from acute exposure to solvents include feelings of intoxication, difficulty in concentrating, and dizziness. Headache, nausea, and vomiting are also known to follow exposure. Chronic lability, depression, and short term memory disturbances, as well as impairments in psychomotor speed, attention, and complex verbal reasoning. This has been referred to in the literature as a psycho–organic syndrome, implying damage to a neural element or from a biochemical disorder in the brain. Psychological tests are more sensitive than clinical medical examinations in detecting early disturbances of the CNS due to solvents [page 6].

The Boeing document comments on specific testing procedures as follows:

[146]

CNS imaging techniques (CT and MRI) are rarely abnormal in neurotoxic disease and are most useful for ruling out other conditions [page 6].

Nerve conduction velocity, electroencephalogram (EEG) in neurotoxic conditions usually disclose only evidence of non-specific axonal dysfunction (diminished amplitude, minimal slowing). For patients complaining of numbness, tingling, or weakness, which are signs of peripheral neuropathy, the NCV test should be performed [page 6].

So far sensory evoked responses use in occupational neurology is limited. By using sensory inputs from the visual, auditory, and somatosensory systems and a computer-averaging technique, the physician can obtain latencies from stimulus to evoked response. Abnormalities of latencies can localize disease in the central and peripheral pathways of these sensory systems [page 7].

The sensory evoked potentials test is a computerized brain map. It has been in use for more than 40 years. It maps electrical activity in the brain following a stimulus (e.g., flashing lights, shock from electrodes, etc.). Like the evoked potentials brain map, other equally valid tests such as the SPECT scan and PET scan are useful for looking at other aspects of the brain — SPECT shows visually the extent to which the brain receives blood; PET shows visually the extent to which the brain uses (metabolizes) nutrients (glucose).

Inclusion of sensory evoked potentials makes it clear that as early as 1989, Seattle-area doctors had knowledge of the evoked potentials brain map. It is highly significant that in no case did an IME referred claimant ever have such a test performed at the request of an IME doctor.

A few more remarks from the Boeing protocol:

Chronic exposure to many neurotoxins may cause disturbances of psychomotor function, deterioration of intellectual capacities, and alteration of emotional stress. [page 8] … Boeing requests a forensic neuro-psychologist be used and that he/she schedule those tests which are deemed appropriate to assess brain impairment [page 9].

This document is so significant because Boeing workers in high numbers began registering chemical injury claims in 1988. Boeing self-administers its workers' compensation program. Boeing workers' compensation program administrators consistently deny these claims. They do so despite the fact that claimants are not given the tests identified in the protocol.

The year 1989 had been a difficult one. By the time OWCP accepted my claim on October 31, I had been without income for ten months. I felt strangled financially. Workers' comp is supposed to be no-fault insurance, but I felt that I had been accused of fraud and had to prove myself not guilty. It appeared to me that OWCP officials were intentionally dragging their feet. I wrote to my Congressman, Rod Chandler. I urged him to break through the red tape and move things along. He did. Suddenly I received checks from the Office of Personnel Management for disability retirement, as well as the severance pay that the Reduction-in-Force (RIF) had made available.

I was unsure what to do. I decided to return the disability retirement and keep the severance pay. Having worked in the personnel department, I knew that severance pay had to be repaid if it was later deemed unwarranted. I also knew that in situations of financial hardship, repayment could be waived. I stumbled along the best I could. After all, I had not yet concluded that the disability was such that eventually I might not work again.

Finally, late in 1989, I did begin receiving compensation checks. Reimbursement for medical expenses, however, proved to be another story altogether.

1990

Early in 1990, chemical sensitives in Washington State got their first "ink on paper" recognition from the state legislature. The campaign to get disabled parking for chemical sensitives had resulted in a hearing, which in turn produced House Bill 2842. The State House passed the bill by unanimous vote on February 9, 1990. Eighteen days later the Senate also passed the bill; again the vote was unanimous. It was signed into law on March 13 and would become effective on June 7, 1990.

Ironically, even as the state government extended this recognition to MCS victims, a doctor at the University of Washington initiated a series of events that would have profoundly damaging effects on how the chemically injured were treated by other government departments. The doctor was the author of the paper "Psychiatric Perspectives on MCSS," which he had presented at the May 1989 occupational medicine conference. This doctor essentially wrote the company line that OWCP had begun to follow, which held that chemical sensitivity syndrome was not a disease but the result of behavioral conditioning, "masked" psychiatric illness, somatization, or hypochondriasis. The study he began in February 1990 would result in a series of medical papers that would perpetuate the company line, increasing the difficulty MCS victims faced in substantiating their workers' compensation claims. Yet this study, like all the papers it produced, was fundamentally flawed.*

On February 14, 1990, I received a letter from this doctor, inviting me to participate in the study. The letter indicated the following:

    1. participation required about an hour, and participants would agree to have blood drawn

    2. information would be kept private (not released to doctors, government agencies, insurance companies, or other outside agencies without participant permission)

    3. MCS patients would be compared with a group of people who were exposed to chemicals but did not get sick

Although I had a lot of reservations, I agreed to participate. I already knew what the doctor was teaching; now I wanted to know what he was doing. I participated early in the process. On the first day of patient examination I was present when the doctor who had provided the patient names showed a folder to the chief researcher. The doctor explained that the folder contained three lists: one group of patients he was sure had MCS; one group of patients he was sure did not have MCS; and a third group that was a toss-up. He told the chief researcher he was eager to see the results of the testing to compare his data with the study doctors'.

What I most remember about the study is a brief neuro-psychological exam conducted by one of the doctors involved. At one point he showed me drawings, then turned them over. After some time had passed, he asked me to draw the set from memory. I could see the drawings right through the paper. I told him that was cheating, because I could see them. I asked him to write on my paper that I cheated, since I'd been able to see them. He assured me that it didn't matter that I saw the drawings.

Following the testing, I wrote the senior author a letter stating my

---

The papers based on this study, as well as other papers mentioned in this chapter, are examined in more detail in Chapter 7. It is interesting to consider them within the timeline of my experience, since the papers and their authors had an influence on how state policy was developing at the time. Readers looking for more information on these papers are invited to turn to Chapter 7.

concerns that the study was biased. I had discussed the "exam" with others and we had compiled a list of numerous indications of bias. The letter included a Freedom of Information request for the source of funding for the study.

On March 20, 1990, the doctor called me back. The funding, he told me, came from the Department of Environmental Health at the University of Washington and from State Labor and Industries. This would turn out to be only part of the truth. (When the paper on the study was published in 1993, the funding acknowledgment read, "University of Washington Department of Environmental Health and the International Association of Machinists/Boeing Health and Safety Institute.") The doctor agreed with me that the study had real problems. He told me that if I'd get the funding, he'd do the study right. He said he was under great pressure to publish and that he hoped to make this study last for 10 years — even though he admitted to me that he knew the study was full of holes and had obvious areas of bias.

Meanwhile I had begun to suspect that OWCP's acceptance of my claim was a fluke — an accident that happened when OWCP officials were caught off guard by the reports of their own doctors. Now those officials seemed to be backpedaling. Not only had I not received reimbursement for medical expenses, but I received a letter from OWCP indicating that they were sending someone out to my home to be sure that everything was going well with my claim. This sounded suspiciously unlike anything I'd ever known a federal agency to do, so I called my attorney. He verified my assumption that OWCP was sending out an investigator.

My attorney was present when the investigator arrived. After about 10 minutes of tension, the investigator admitted to my attorney the reason for the visit. Afterward my attorney requested by the Freedom of Information Act a copy of the investigation. The report indicated that OWCP was in fact giving me a hard time. It seemed to me to be an exorbitant waste of money to do such an investigation. I was just one little person in the Pacific Northwest. When I considered the other chemically injured workers in the state and nationwide, I wondered how any workers' compensation program could justify the expense, assuming this were a routine practice.

If I needed further proof that OWCP wanted me off the rolls, it soon arrived in the form of another letter. This time, OWCP informed me that they had arranged for me to have several independent medical exams (IMEs). I was to see an allergist, a pulmonologist, and a psychiatrist. These appointments were arranged through a consulting group — a group whose name I recognized all too well, since I knew they had set up most of the IMEs for chemically injured Boeing workers. Those workers' claims were routinely rejected. There was little reason to doubt OWCP's intent.

This consulting group is a conglomerate of sorts. They contract with certain doctors to perform IMEs for workers' compensation administrators. Their written objective is to provide exams independent of employee or employer. However, the consulting group, like any other business, needs to make money. Any consultant of value knows exactly what the preferred outcome is for any consulting effort. For workers' comp programs, the value of such consultants is their ability to locate doctors likely to support their objectives for claims denial. That way, bureaucrats are less likely to be seen as "doctor shopping."

That may seem like a radical accusation, but consider the structure of the "consultant" operations. A normal doctor-patient relationship is one to one. Everything is confidential unless the patient agrees otherwise. Payment comes from the patient. In contrast, an IME doctor's responsibility is not to the patient; it is to the patient's employer or workers' comp department, other government agencies (e.g., Social Security), or the patient's opponents in litigation. The doctor sends the report to those paying for it, not to the patient. IMEs are also called defense exams.

The consulting group that arranged my exams had several rules by which patients were expected to abide — rules that represent an alarming departure from standard medical practice. Perhaps the most significant is that the patient is to have no contact with the doctor after leaving the exam. The patient cannot see the report and has no way to deal with the doctor to correct errors or misrepresentations. As the patient is shuffled from one IME to another, such errors can grow by leaps and bounds. Other problems arising from IME doctors' refusal to deal with patients after the IME exam will become clear later.

My appointments with the doctors selected by the consulting group were all on the same day, April 20, 1990. They were all in the same area downtown in Seattle. By this time I knew that air downtown was a real problem for me. Treating doctors had made it clear that I needed to avoid downtown or any location with moderate to heavy traffic. One of the explanations was that "brain fog" is evidence of brain destruction. When neurons are struggling, they consume great volumes of oxygen. Heavy traffic further reduces available oxygen, and the exhaust contributes to "brain fog."

[151]

I took a taxi downtown rather than chance driving with "brain fog." I saw the allergist, then the psychiatrist, then the pulmonologist. I remember very little of what took place. (I took notes between sessions or I'd remember nothing.) It took me a while to find the pulmonologist's office. I was confused at that point. I had been inside tight buildings, which are a problem, and being in the dirty air of downtown contributed to the confusion. I was struggling. My only clear memories of that day are from the pulmonologist's office, where I had to sit on an elevated piece of furniture. There were no rails or walls for support. I was seeing too many images of the same thing and was nauseated and dizzy. My ears rang like crazy. (Most of the time my ear ringing is like a computer hum. When I am exposed to substances that bother me, it's more like a tea kettle whistle.) The doctor kept coming in and out of the room. He would be gone for long periods of time, during which I'd try to steady myself. Finally I'd get down from the height and sit on the foot rest of the elevated table. When he came back in, I'd climb back up. This happened over and over. I wanted to grab him and tell him to stay until the end of the exam, but I would not have known which one of him to grab.

On a different day I had to return to the allergist's to have blood drawn so he could send it for testing to a university in the Midwest. I had to return to a hospital twice for the pulmonologist to test my breathing on an exercise test and with a methacholine challenge.

The initial trip made me sick. The return visits made me even sicker. What came from two of the return visits only added injury to insult.

The methacholine challenge came first. I don't know why the doctor felt a need to administer this test. He had my medical record. Six doctors had diagnosed asthma. Before I went to the hospital for that testing, I called the pulmonologist's office and asked whether any people had ever had adverse reactions to methacholine. I was assured that the answer was no. I waited a day or two, called and asked the same question, and received the same answer. I went for testing.

The irony here is that the exam is set up to bring about a response of asthma. Instead of a challenge with a smelly carpet, they were using a substance that was new to me. I knew what a carpet would do. I didn't know what methacholine (provocholine) would do. I had done a little research, but all I learned was that the drug had been tested on monkeys, not people.

Prior to the test my asthma level was mild. Following the administration of methacholine, my asthma level reached a new level of moderate.

The change in level was permanent. I was outraged. The doctor had my medical record. He knew that I had systemic reactions to all antibiotics at this point. He knew that I could not tolerate bronchodilators with freon propellants, nor could I tolerate oral steroids. That spells sensitivity. Yet he decided to perform the methacholine challenge anyway.

The exercise test was scheduled for another day. It seemed to me an unjustifiable expense, since nowhere in my records was there any indication that exercise and asthma were thought to be linked. Nevertheless, I traveled downtown once again. The doctor arrived late for the 9:00 A.M. test. The technician told me it was obvious that the doctor would have preferred doing the test at another time, but I did not intend to reschedule.

The doctor had a lot of difficulty finding the blood vessel. He stabbed and stabbed. The female technician turned white and kept looking away. The doctor kept grumbling that this wasn't the best time for this test. He wanted to stop and reschedule. I just wanted to get it done. It was a fairly gory mess. At my elbow and wrist there were large watery lumps oozing blood all over the place. Blood ran down my arm, through my fingers, and all over the floor.

After the test the doctor wanted to know what I remembered. I told him my legs hurt. During the test I had had to ride a bicycle. Later, evoked potentials testing would show that the effort was greater than the post-test comments by the technicians on the data sheets, which were "excellent effort" and "test terminated due to leg fatigue." Had they been able to guess what the effort took after the ride downtown and the experience in the tight hospital building, they would have been surprised.

As for myself, I was surprised at the damage done by a totally unnecessary test. The circumference of my right and left arms made my arms appear to belong to two different people.

Later, I discovered a terrible truth: This pulmonologist had seen a chemically sensitive patient several months before he saw me. That person had an adverse reaction to the methacholine challenge. He saw another months after he saw me. That person had the same experience. Because the consultant group refuses to let patients contact a doctor after an IME, the doctor is insulated from the knowledge that he has done damage, and may do damage again. This is unconscionable.

In case this sounds like something dreamed up, I did ask to have pictures the evening following the exercise test. The zombie-like look is just "brain fog" after the experience with indoor and outdoor pollution.

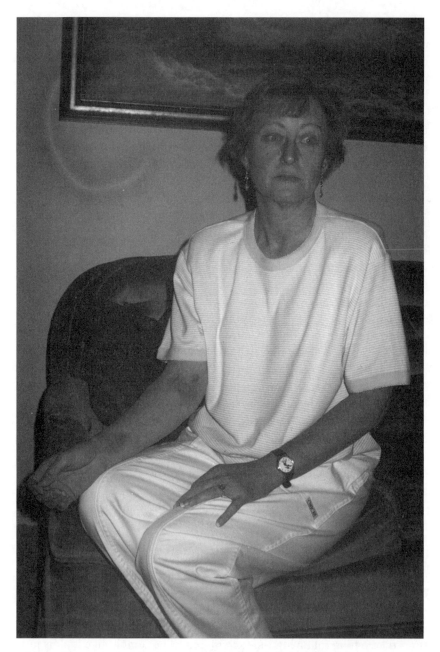

The author one day after her appointment with the IME pulmonologist.

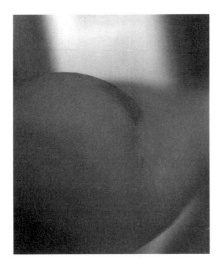

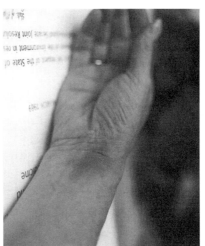

Top, left: Artery search site by elbow. Note swollen tissue. *Top, right:* Artery search site — wrist. Note multiple punctures. *Bottom, right:* Artery search site by elbow. Note multiple punctures.

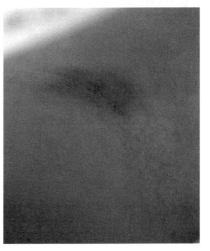

Presumably all the doctors I saw through the consultant group knew that there were other tests available for the chemically injured. The Boeing corporation routinely used the same consultant group to schedule IMEs, and the doctors I saw had all seen the Boeing IME protocol, which specified appropriate tests. Why did they not run these tests on me — or, indeed, on any of the Boeing workers? Could it be that the employers who pay their bills would prefer *not* to have data that establish brain injury — and the doctors know it? One thing is certain: If a doctor neglects to perform meaningful tests, he won't get meaningful data.

It is instructive to look through an issue of a publication put out by the consultant group that set up my appointments. *Issues of Injury*, Volume 8, number 3, features a front-page article titled "The Chemically Sensitive" (http://www.mcn.com/ioi/1994/mcs.htm). Page 2 of this article includes a cartoon of a fat woman, hands on hips and clothespin on nose. A tag line on page 3 of the article announces, "Mass illness can be created more easily by suggestion and incentive than by any chemical or biological agent." A new article on page 4 is entitled "Multiple chemical sensitivity MAPPING A DEFENSE." (Use of upper and lower case letters is the way the title is set.) The article is available at http://www.mcn.com/ioi/1994/MCSLEGAL.HTM. Finally, on the back cover where the magazine is folded, just under and to the left of the address, is a clue to the articles inside: "Multiple Chemical Sensitivity: Medically Suspect, Politically Correct." This from a group that purports to provide nonbiased exams.

The general public has no idea that state and federal taxes support such consultants and the doctors they hire. By the time I found out, I was beyond outrage. Instead, I felt an overwhelming sadness. I knew the chemically injured. Two local people, unable to handle the stress of their illness, were dead by their own hand. One comment often used by IME doctors is "Nobody ever died of MCS"—but I knew two. A person who has taken the task of documenting suicides among the chemically injured has compiled a list of nearly 100 instances nationwide. Could it be that the known suicides are but an ice crystal on the tip of the iceberg?

Throughout 1990 I had been in touch with my U.S. congressman, Rod Chandler, and Senator Brock Adams. After the IMEs I was attempting to generate interest for a hearing on the OWCP treatment of chemically injured federal workers. Rod Chandler assured me that if I could produce numbers of similarly injured workers, a hearing would be quite likely. At a personal level, I also wanted reimbursement for medical expenses. OWCP's response was that if I'd quit talking to my congressman, I might get reimbursed.

Just after the appointments with the IME doctors, I had an appointment in Portland, Oregon, to see a clinical neuropsychologist. The psychiatrist I had chosen to see had referred me. The doctor was associated with Dr. Muriel Lezak, author of *Neurological Assessment*, 2d ed. (Oxford University Press, 1983). Authority of the findings should be without question.

Up to that point I had been rather optimistic that somehow, someday, I'd improve and return to work. I tried to make my brain relearn how to deal with numbers. I did this often. I wasn't having any success, but I assumed that eventually that might change. The findings from that neuropsychological exam, however, gave me pause. It was apparent that my optimism was unfounded. Test results showed:

[156]

99 percentile on high school vocabulary

average to high vocabulary and fund of knowledge

premorbid intellectual ability in high average range

average to high average on visual analysis of missing elements in
pictures

normal limits on visual organization

impaired attention and concentration

moderately to severely impaired on psychomotor speed, mental
tracking and visual scanning

learning and memory compromised

low average visual memory

language intact

conceptualization intact

impaired on test of distractibility — this test reflects ability to
inhibit responses in the face of competing stimuli — she performed in the 6th percentile

not overly symptom focused

The summary of findings stated that "Ms. Matthews demonstrated
moderate to severe attentional deficits and moderate to severe learning and
memory deficits. Old learned verbal skills, visuospatial abilities, language,
and conceptual functions appear intact. These findings are consistent with
chemical exposure.... I would estimate her overall impairment level to be
in the moderate range."

This information was disquieting. The picture was worse than I had
thought. That I might score in the sixth percentile in anything blew my
mind.

On July 19, 1990, *The American Journal of Psychiatry* published "Allergic to Life: Psychological Factors in Environmental Illness." It expressed
the bias: "psychologic vulnerability influences chemical sensitivity following chemical exposure." I do not use the term bias loosely. One of the
authors had served on a panel in 1988 to disprove that chemically injured
Boeing workers had real problems; following that she continued to receive
Boeing workers as IME patients. The Boeing IME protocol told her what
to test for, but she did not run any of the tests indicated. Her lack of action
violates a medical principle: rule out all physical problems before considering psychiatric factors. A further expression of the article's bias is the
title; it pokes fun at a patient group, which is unprofessional.

[157]

IV : Personal Experience with MCS

In July 1990 the *Western Journal of Medicine* published "An Outbreak of Illness Among Aerospace Workers." The senior author was the doctor mentioned above, and the second listed author was the one conducting the study in which I'd participated in February. This article, like the one just described, dwelled on "psychiatric disorders" and "psychosocial factors." Clearly the doctor who had done the February study was biased. Even as he claimed to be conducting important research, he was being published expressing his preconceptions.

Meanwhile, a friend I'd encouraged to participate in that terrible study was told by his workers' comp program that they would take no further action on his case until they could obtain the results of his participation in the study. This was evidence that information about the study and the participants had been leaked. Indeed, the protection which participants were assured of in the invitational letter proved to be as full of holes as a colander. A deposition pointed to "Boeing company attorneys' inappropriate and unauthorized use of findings from the UW Multiple Chemical Sensitivity Study." Were study findings leaked to Boeing because they were partly paying for the study? The International Association of Machinists/Boeing Health and Safety Institute receives money for such purposes from the employer, Boeing.

As the year progressed I became frustrated by OWCP's refusal to pay medical expenses which, having accepted my claim, they were required to pay. Thousands of dollars were ignored. The lead bill pay examiner assured me in June that my bills would be paid. I had sent a folder of carefully organized receipts and other documents, hoping that the material would not become lost. In September 1990 my attorney received a letter from a manager at OWCP stating, "I regret that the organized folder of bills provided by Ms. Matthews June 25 did not reach the attention of our lead bill pay examiner"— naming the same person who had signed the letter of June 25 promising payment! Those bills have never been paid.

There was further OWCP activity in September. Having sent me to IME doctors to establish a conflict of medical opinion, OWCP now informed me that a "referee exam" was necessary to resolve the conflict. The letter invited Mr. Sweeting to submit names of impartial medical examiners. Mr. Sweeting suggested Dr. B —, who is board-certified in family medicine. Cuff notes from my OWCP file (which Mr. Sweeting obtained from my file) show a flurry of activity as case workers tried to determine Dr. B —'s credentials.

[158]

During the end of October and the first part of November an OWCP doctor assured my attorney that OWCP had selected Dr. B — as the referee and that he had approval to tell me to go ahead and make an appointment with Dr. B. I called the doctor, explaining that OWCP had told me to make an appointment and that the purpose was to referee a conflict. Neither the doctor's office nor I heard anything further from OWCP. A letter from the doctor's office to OWCP, dated November 5, 1990, is contained in my OWCP file. The letter states that I was booked for a November 13 appointment. A handwritten note on the letter reads, "Let this exam go forward." It is initialed by an OWCP employee.

I kept the appointment, and no one heard from OWCP. On December 6, 1990, Dr. B — sent a preliminary report to OWCP stating:

> Bonnye Matthews has Multiple Chemical Sensitivity Syndrome (MCSS), Organic Brain Syndrome, and occupational induced asthma. These illnesses were caused by exposure to toxic chemicals at work when carpet and glues were added to her building environment.... Her prognosis is poor as there is no known cure.... She does not need any further testing to document her impairments. In fact, to do further testing would be detrimental to her health.

As the year ended, I felt I had really been through the wringer, but I thought that things were turning around and the stressful ordeal with OWCP was about to come to a fitting end. I was trying to deal with the likelihood that I would not be able to return to work. It was still very difficult to imagine, and the loss of mental ability was painful. I was working hard to locate chemically injured federal workers all across the United States. They provided me with information and support. I also had a very supportive family, and a sense of hope that seemed to be indomitable.

1991

Less than a month into the new year, I discovered that my hope was unfounded. I had still not heard anything from OWCP regarding Dr. B —'s report, so my attorney wrote to inquire whether the case would now move forward. A few days later (Feb. 1, 1991), I received a letter from OWCP stating that I had been scheduled for a February 14 appointment with still another doctor. "There is a conflict in medical opinion in your file and this impartial physician(s) is being selected to resolve the conflict," OWCP wrote.

I was dumbfounded. This letter was signed by the very same OWCP doctor who had told my attorney that I should go ahead and make an appointment with Dr. B — for the referee exam. The Federal Employees' Compensation Act had no provision for *two* referee exams. Even more disturbing was the name of the doctor that OWCP was insisting I see. She was the doctor whose authorship of the 1990 papers "Allergic to Life" and "An Outbreak of Illness Among Aerospace Workers" had helped establish the belief that the symptoms of chemically injured workers were largely due to psychiatric disorders or psychosocial factors. This was the unbiased doctor to whom OWCP was entrusting my case!

I was still naive enough to believe it was possible to discuss concerns in a reasonable manner with people at OWCP, so I called. The telephone conversations were recorded in my OWCP file. First, the person I spoke to wrote a note to a claims examiner, describing my call:

> Why is she being referred out again. She has no response from her evaluation by Dr. B —, which she considers a ref. opinion. She wants some answers…. Her appointment is February 14. She wants it changed. I told her I would not change it until you spoke with her & you tell me to change it.

The claims examiner phoned me to respond. His note reads:

> I called and explained Dr. B was not an IME. The appt was set up by either her or her attorney and he did not have benefit of a SOAF [statement of accepted fact] or the medical evidence of record. IME has been scheduled….

What the claims examiner failed to record is the sheer nastiness of his call. I have never had anyone taunt me like he did. I wanted truth and a simple explanation. Instead I received intense verbal abuse. The examiner literally laughed and sneered at me for thinking Dr. B — was a referee. I tried to explain that I had no intention of seeing another doctor, since the referee exam with Dr. B — had been OWCP's idea. The examiner laughed. He told me that regardless of what the circumstances may have been, I could never prove that Dr. B — had been a referee. He told me it was his goal to get me off the rolls, and I couldn't do a thing about it. For the first time in my life, I hung up the receiver on another person while he was speaking. From that point until this day I have not talked directly with anyone at OWCP. My attorney has handled all communication.

We now know, but did not know at the time, that a letter dated February 4, 1991, went from OWCP to their chosen "referee" doctor: "We are sending you the case of Bonnye L. Matthews for examination and opinion … for resolving a conflict in medical opinion…. Enclosed is a statement dated February 13, 1990, which presents the accepted facts in this case." It is important to note that the date, 2/13/90, is prior to the date of the doctor appointments arranged by the consulting group — the appointments that supposedly created the conflict in medical opinion. It is also worth noting that although the OWCP was supposed to have provided me a statement of accepted fact (SOAF) prior to IME appointments. I never received one.

In their letter to the second referee doctor, OWCP added this: "NOTE: Please refer Ms. Matthews to a Psychiatrist and an Allergist after you have seen her." What is important to note here is that OWCP is supposed to select doctors for referral themselves. The selection is supposed to be random. For them to have asked an IME doctor for a referral is inappropriate.

Strange things must have been occurring at OWCP. My attorney told me that the OWCP doctor with whom he had corresponded had asked him to mail Dr. B—'s curriculum vitae to the doctor's home address. On February 6, 1991, after Mr. Sweeting had made it clear that OWCP had chosen a biased doctor in the second referee selection, the OWCP doctor asked to see a videotape in which the OWCP-selected referee makes it clear what her position on chemical sensitivity is. The tape is titled *Canary Blues* and was produced by Alphonse Doce. Mr. Sweeting asked me to mail the copy to the doctor's home, since the doctor had told Mr. Sweeting that if it went to OWCP, he might not receive it.

I viewed all this with no little consternation. My attorney requested in writing that OWCP respond to his allegation of bias on the part of the referee. A formal decision should have been forthcoming from OWCP prior to my attending the appointment. If they concluded she was not biased, I should have been given appeal rights prior to keeping the appointment.

OWCP cuff notes from February 12 and 13, 1991, are revealing. Another claims examiner — not the one who harassed me on the phone — writes:

> phone call to Dennis Mankin, N.O., Director FEC — Mankin spoke with Markey re: issue of giving a formal decision. Per Markey, *do not* issue appeal rights on issue of bias.

[161]

A second note to the file from the same examiner:

> I called D. Mankin back & pointed out Chap —[writing unclear] 3-500
> pg 6 — specifically states a formal denial may be issued if requested by clmt
> (Sect 4 pg 6). He acknowledged it said that, & change will be forthcom-
> ing. Meanwhile, OK to issue decision, but not w/ appeal rts.

"Markey" presumably was Thomas Markey, at that time the second
in command at OWCP headquarters. Decisions regarding claims made by
federally injured workers are supposed to be made at the district level, not
at headquarters. What my file documents is that a very high level official
in Washington, D.C., was making decisions for the handling of my case —
and possibly even fiddling with the rules to accommodate his actions.

What Seattle district officials chose to do was nothing. They simply
never ruled on the issue of bias. Meanwhile, I had to make a decision about
this "referee" appointment. My treating physicians had repeatedly warned
me that I should not go into the downtown area. OWCP had scheduled the
appointment at morning rush hour, and there were two large conventions
in Seattle on that date. Traffic would be a nightmare. If I failed to keep the
appointment, however, OWCP would be able to remove me immediately for
what they called "obstruction."

It was one of those "damned if you do and damned if you don't" situations. I did not wish to make removing me any easier or more inexpen-
sive than necessary for OWCP. Disregarding the advice of all my doctors, I
kept the appointment.

Once again, I took a taxi. It was no surprise that we were held up in
traffic. By the time I reached the second referee's office building I was experiencing the disorientation that comes from "brain fog." I had trouble seeing. Dizziness was overcoming me. When I entered the office building, I
immediately encountered a woman wearing perfume. That added to the
difficulty. I pulled upon every part of my being to hold together. My fear
was that I might collapse and be hospitalized. To me survival meant avoiding the hospital, especially under the care of the doctor I was about to see.

I have little spots of memory of that visit. Since OWCP refuses to permit anyone to take any other person into a referee exam, I remember asking if I could record the exam on audio tape. I explained that she'd remember
what happened but that I would not be able to. The doctor grudgingly
agreed.

The audio tape makes it perfectly clear that I told this doctor I was experiencing organic brain syndrome. I told her not once, but three or four times. Furthermore, my medical records make it perfectly clear that organic brain syndrome is part of my medical history since the poisoning at work. She did not know me, but my having told her should have caused her to take care. She ignored me each time I told her. The audio tape also shows that she told me she had not read my case file prior to the visit.

Her exam was superficial. At one point in the checklist she used, there is a note that she checked for a deviated septum. Her finding was negative. An ear, nose, throat specialist who saw me later had no difficulty seeing a deviated septum. I say this not because the deviated septum was significant to the issue before her, but because it raises questions about the attention she devoted to my exam. Could it be that the exam was designed not to see anything? Certainly she did not perform any of the tests outlined in the Boeing IME protocol, even though as a consultant to Boeing she had to have been familiar with the document — had perhaps even helped to write it. Any of those tests would have been appropriate for my case.

That visit produced the worst health effect to date. It can best be summed up by reports from the doctors I saw, trying to get the reaction turned around.

From family physician, February 21, 1991:

> I am today witnessing a severe reaction she has since going into downtown Seattle, 5 days ago, and being required to stay for some time in an air tight building and being exposed to perfume as well as probably other chemicals to which she is sensitive.
>
> The most disturbing part of her presentation today is a definite clouded sensorium. This was witnessed also yesterday by telephone. She is having some difficulty expressing herself — a situation never seen in her before. She also still has the dry frequent cough she usually demonstrates with exposure.

From clinical psychologist, February 22, 1991:

> This was a neuropsychological assessment to determine whether there was any difference between the findings of May 1989 and the current situation. The difference essentially was a loss of IQ from 115 to 98. [A year later, testing would prove that the deterioration was permanent.]

From psychiatrist after review of the report from clinical psychologist, March 11, 1991:

> With my previous diagnosis of an organic brain syndrome secondary to chemical exposure and to multiple chemical sensitivity ... it is my recommendation that this patient not be subjected to any more testing that involves her exposure to chemicals, and that any evaluations of her ... must be accomplished in arenas which are as chemical free as is possible, which definitely does not include the downtown Seattle area, its confines, or most of the medical buildings therein.
>
> This letter might appear sterile but is ... an indication of the clear deterioration that this patient has undergone because of her multiple chemical sensitivity and continued re-exposures .... [T]o force this individual to be exposed, in my estimation, is negligence.

From clinical neuropsychologist, March 22, 1991:

> level of impairment now is classified in the **severely impaired** range

For some time after the exam by OWCP's second referee, my attorney battled with OWCP. OWCP claimed that this referee felt she needed to refer me out to an allergist and psychiatrist. Yet it was clear that OWCP directed her to do that in their letter to her written 10 days before my appointment. When I discovered that more exams were planned and that they were downtown, I told my attorney I would not go. I was too badly damaged. OWCP pointed out that my refusal to keep the appointments could be considered "obstruction," which could result in my being removed from the rolls. But I didn't intend to die or end up in a nursing home from keeping OWCP's appointments.

I was totally unable to follow what was happening, though Mr. Sweeting kept me informed. My disorientation lasted for weeks. When Mr. Sweeting discovered the results of the damage from that one visit, he planned to file a tort claim.

Interestingly enough, Thomas Morgan, director of the Seattle District Office of OWCP, wrote to my attorney in a letter dated March 1, 1991:

> We will give your client a formal decision on our finding that [the doctor] is not biased, and that she was properly selected to perform this examination. If she disagrees with this decision she can exercise her right of appeal.

The formal decision never came, yet this letter seems to serve the purpose without appeal rights as ordered by headquarters. Why Thomas Morgan wrote this is unclear. Thomas Markey at OWCP in Washington, D.C., had ordered Seattle not to issue appeal rights if they ruled on bias.

On March 6, 1991, Mr. Sweeting wrote to the U.S. Department of Labor, ESA/OWCP Branch of Hearings & Review, that we were appealing the decision that the referee was not biased.

An OWCP employee's cuff notes dated March 4, 1991, state:

> [Referee doctor's] office mailed the rept & case file back to us on Fri, Mar 1 per phone call from [a claims examiner] saying he needed the report ASAP. He [Mr. Sweeting] also questioned why "I" am referring her to an Allergist & Psych. I am not referring her to any doctors. In our original letter to [the referee] this office asked her to make these referrals.

This is just another piece of evidence that OWCP, rather than the doctor had requested the referrals, even though they told my attorney otherwise.

This note also brings up the fact that when OWCP refers a person to a doctor, they send the case file to the doctor's office. In an age of automation, it is very surprising that the OWCP has a paper case file system. That unique, unphotocopied file actually leaves the office. Had there been a fire in the doctor's office, OWCP would have lost my entire file, which was quite large. For that matter, how does OWCP determine that nothing has been lost while the file was in a doctor's custody? One thing, however, is clear: Having a single file enables OWCP to claim that they cannot pay bills while files are elsewhere (e.g., at IME doctor offices).

As for the second referee doctor's report, it read as follows:

> Ms. Matthews describes symptoms in multiple organ systems that she attributes to low level exposures to a variety of chemically and biologically unrelated substances. This syndrome is not likely to be related to any specific workplace exposures while working for the Army Corps of Engineers, more probably than not. Psychiatric factors which may predispose her to the development of such symptoms have been alluded to by other examiners. Ms. Matthews is engaged full time in the perpetuation of her explanatory model for the above symptoms. There is a great deal of outside reinforcement for this activity. It is very unlikely that she will return to continuous employment in her former position.

Evidently she did get around to reading my file at some point, since she refers to the reports of other doctors; her wording, however, is interesting. She does not state that she found "psychiatric factors" in her examination, only that others have "alluded" (implied or indirectly referred) to them. This sentence is neither a conclusion nor a diagnosis. It only refers to information that OWCP already had in their file. It resolves no conflict.

Presumably being "engaged full time in the perpetuation of her explanatory model for the above symptoms" meant that I was writing a book. (Again, this information must have come from my file, since I did not mention the book to the doctor.) Actually, in my research and writing I was not seeking to "perpetuate" anything about my symptoms; I was gathering information that I thought would be useful to other people in my situation. (OWCP consistently interpreted my book writing as evidence that my workers' compensation claim was somehow false or deceptive; apparently they assumed that if I could write a book, I had suffered no brain damage. They ignored the fact that testing showed predominant damage to math skills rather than verbal abilities.)

When the doctor writes, "She attributes to low level exposures to a variety of chemically and biologically unrelated substances," she glosses over the fact that such attribution was based on the opinions of a large number of doctors. I did not have the capacity to dream all this up. I did not diagnose myself. If this referee believed that the doctors were wrong, she should have said so, and stated why she disagreed with them. Instead, she focused her argument on the only non-medical person — me — by implying that I had diagnosed myself. This kind of argument fails to stand up to scrutiny.

The doctor's report was based on a single exam (lasting about an hour) coupled with her reading of reports, not one of which ever positively identified a psychiatric or psychological problem. After refusing to deal with the question of bias, OWCP accepted the report without regard to the lack of evidence. Another problem with OWCP's acceptance of the report is that the doctor is not board certified in either neurology or psychiatry. OWCP is supposed to use board-certified doctors.

Over and over, OWCP violated their own rules by sending me to this doctor. Another fact that should have disqualified her was her association with the two doctors in occupational medicine to whom I had already been sent by a self-selected pulmonologist; an IME doctor is not supposed to be associated with anyone the patient has already seen. These doctors all worked at institutions affiliated with one another, and the OWCP referee was in the process of writing a paper with one of the occupational medicine doctors I had seen when she saw me.

One thing was certain: If the OWCP had been hoping I would go back to work, their own actions had now prevented that possibility. It might have been possible, before that doctor's exam, for me to have improved enough to someday return to work. After that office visit, there was no longer any chance for that kind of improvement.

On March 4, 1991, my attorney prepared and I signed the tort claim based on the damage subsequent to this doctor's exam. Personal injury: "Severe emotional distress, aggravation of underlying organic brain syndrome, aggravation of multiple chemical sensitivities." On March 6 the tort claim was transmitted with a cover letter from Mr. Sweeting.

On March 12, 1991, Thomas Morgan at OWCP wrote to Mr. Sweeting: "It is standard practice to allow referee medical examiners to utilize consultants from other medical specialties to resolve all questions raised in our Statement of Accepted Facts (SOAF)." (As the OWCP file would later demonstrate, OWCP was not "allowing" Dr. Sparks to make referrals, but requesting that she do so.) The letter continued: "You have previously been advised that Dr. B — did not have the case file or a statement of accepted facts prior to his examination of Ms. Matthews. This diminishes the probative value of his report." OWCP refused to take into consideration the fact that I went to every exam with a complete set of data, which I contended was every bit as valid as OWCP's. After all, I kept mine tightly bound and never left the original anywhere. OWCP had absolutely no way to know whether any of the documents in their file had been lost either at the Harborview–University of Washington exams or the ones they scheduled with the consultant group. Furthermore, the second referee doctor who did have my case file before the requested exam did not read it prior to the exam ... so why was OWCP so insistent on its presence? As for the statement of accepted fact, this was the document (already mentioned) dated *before* the exams that supposedly created the conflict of opinion — a document I had not seen, though OWCP was supposed to have provided it to me, and a statement that contained significant errors.

On March 29, 1991, OWCP cuff notes read:

> RE: B Matthews, A14-240613 Note my telecon of 3/29 — Pls. move to suspend benefits due to obstruction 5 USC 8123 (d). Send a cc of lt. to U.S. Solicitor's Office Attn Paul Klingenberg — He's handling tort claim.

The tort claim has remained a mystery. Some time passed after the claim went forward. My attorney received a call from the office asking for more information. He responded by asking them to specify what information they wanted. Since then the tort claim has been inactive. Perhaps the hope is that it will be forgotten.

Right on the heels of the exam by the OWCP referee, I had an appointment at the University of California at Irvine at the Brain Imaging Center to have a specialized test called the PET scan with the MCS protocol. Essentially they were looking at the brain's uptake of glucose (how the brain is fed) in patients who were diagnosed with multiple chemical sensitivity. This appointment was based on a referral by a neurologist/psychiatrist in Montana who had experience with these cases. I had searched for a neurologist in Washington State and been unable to find one who seemed knowledgeable about chemical injury. (Was it possible that doctors in Washington were experiencing some pressure not to deal with the MCSS issue?)

This trip to the Brain Imaging Center would provide even more concrete evidence that the symptoms I identified were not something I dreamed up because I didn't want to face a psychiatric diagnosis but rather were completely understandable in terms of actual brain damage and resultant dysfunction.

The tests showed three brain lesions: one in the right temporal region, one on the left located at the uncus, and the third on the left in the hippocampus. With the brain damage I had, new learning was difficult. I had studied hard to understand the immunological aspects of MCS. Neurology was an entirely new field.

I also saw the doctor in Montana who had referred me to the Brain Imaging Center. He concluded that the brain damage was significant, and he assured me that the PET scan from California clearly supported this finding. OWCP passed off his reports as if they were irrelevant. This doctor, who had experience with OWCP at another district level, was not surprised. His letter of June 28, 1991, states:

> With regard to specific findings with respect to toxic encephalopathy in your case, there is certainly evidence on the PET scanning that there is a low-grade organic mental syndrome associated with memory defects, seen both on the psychometric as well as your PET scan with reduction in glucose metabolism in the hippocampal region which is indeed the area of the brain most associated with memory.
>
> In view of the combination of the organic injury to the nervous system, organic mental syndrome, memory defects, chemical sensitivities which you have already documented ... there appears to be no chance that you will be able to work in any capacity that I can visualize. Therefore, the final diagnosis as seen now is a combination of chemical sensitivities as well

as toxic encephalopathy. Without much question this will be, with a high probability, a permanent state of affairs.

The OWCP made much of the "low-grade" terminology in the above letter, and in a letter to me dated December 30, 1991, the neurologist/psychiatrist explains:

> Basically what we have said or at least have tried to say is that you do not have large area defects, i.e., total temporal lobe, frontal lobe, parietal lobe damage with evidence of huge areas of the brain being affected by the metabolic defects that we talked about in the hippocampus and medial temporal region. Since these were areas that were relatively small in volume size, that is the reason we use the word minimal. However, that does not excuse the idea that it is, in fact, in the same area that one would expect it to be to have caused memory defects. ... described as being severe, and that stands on its own feet. It does not compare in any sense to the metabolic functioning that we have talked about in the PET scan, only in so far as they both point to the same area of the brain as being abnormal and it doesn't mean ... that significant damage has not been done. This is simply another gymnastic episode in the thinking of bureaucratic people at the Work Comp level that you don't have anything wrong with you.

Just after the appointment in California, I received a letter from OWCP dated April 5, 1991. It was another threat to remove me from compensation for not attending the additional exams. The letter stated that I had 15 days to explain why the appointments were canceled.

The tort claim had been filed March 6, 1991. As I received medical reports from doctors who assessed the damage subsequent to the referee exam, I sent those reports to Matt. Matt sent them immediately to OWCP, who therefore should have had no question about why I did not attend any more medical appointments downtown. OWCP was still maintaining that the doctor had a need for additional medical referrals, when all along it was OWCP who inappropriately told her to make those referrals.

On April 9, my attorney responded to Thomas Morgan, director of OWCP Seattle District. One paragraph states:

> We continue to feel that your claim handling is designed to intentionally harass Ms. Matthews. We have submitted numerous medical opinions indicating that Ms. Matthews cannot venture into the downtown Seattle area without suffering further cognitive impairment, and therefore it is unreasonable to ask that she go to any further examinations in the area. To ignore these reports only proves the intentional nature of your concerted effort to harm Ms. Matthews.

[169]

IV : Personal Experience with MCS

My file contains a record of a phone call made by an OWCP case examiner to the Employees Compensation Appeal Board (ECAB) on April 12, 1991:

> ECAB requested case and I called to advise there is no appealable decision. I spoke with T — who said atty was appealing 3/1/91 letter. I read it to her and we agreed it was not a formal decision. I will fax appropriate documents ... she will have docket canceled.

OWCP had played games with the issue of formal decision on bias. They had created a letter (March 1, 1991) *after* the appointment had been kept stating that they would give me a decision, but they had never actually issued the decision, presumably to prevent appeal rights. My attorney decided to use the March 1 letter as the basis for his March 6 appeal, since OWCP refused to write the formal decision on bias with appeal rights.

In all the disorientation following the second referee exam, the discomfort following the trip to California and back, and the frustration that comes when the discovery is made that the issue isn't one of logic and reason but rather secret intent and clear wrongdoing, stress increased.

It was also stressful to realize, as I now did, that officials in high levels of government, who might have been able to put things right, were not interested in extending their hands to help. The corruption of the letter and spirit of the Federal Employees Compensation Act and its effect on chemically injured federal workers throughout the country had stirred not a ripple on the waters of the Congress or the executive branch. Members of the House and Senate, as well as the president, had received complaints from chemically injured federal workers all over the country. This was not a party issue. Members of the Republican and Democratic parties responded the same way. They would contact the Department of Labor. The action would be relayed to OWCP headquarters, who would deny that there was any problem. Then a copy of the letter from headquarters would be sent to the injured worker, and that was the end of that. Consequently, chemically injured workers all over the country were sick, becoming increasingly impoverished, and generally were frustrated that others in federal service were going to add to the numbers. No one appeared to care to investigate. Without oversight, OWCP could do as it pleased. The longer the lack of oversight lasted, the worse the problem was likely to become.

The Reagan administration and its cost-cutting measures — which eliminated oversight functions — could be credited with much of the problem. During that time, those of us at the Office of Personnel Management realized that the personnel management oversight that had held many federal agencies in check against employee abuse had been terminated with the Civil Service Reform Act. We wondered what effect that might have on programs and employees in the future. Now I was finding out.

My recognition that chemical sensitives were being deprived of government redress affected me profoundly, for it affected the manner in which I framed my hope that right would prevail. I could not really bring myself to believe that my case would never be put right, but I did realize that it might take more than an act of Congress.

On April 12, 1991, Mr. Sweeting sent the following to OWCP:

> Attached please find a handwritten note from my client, Ms. Matthews, dated 4-8-91. We have previously submitted reports from doctor (four listed) regarding the unreasonableness of asking Ms. Matthews to be examined in the downtown Seattle area. As you can see, your failure to heed earlier medical reports has resulted in an increased neuropsychological impairment. My client is frustrated, confused, and frightened by the tactics utilized by your staff. Please advise as to any further action you intend to take.

On July 10, 1991, Matt sent a letter transmitting the medical reports from the neurologist/psychiatrist with the PET scan color picture of the brain damage. He mentioned that the doctor had indicated that I was "unable to work and that this is a permanent condition."

With a letter dated September 9, 1991, I received from OWCP the notice of termination. Interestingly, "obstruction" was not the reason. (This plan had apparently been dropped somewhere along the way, with a note that the second referee had indicated she did not need the exams by the other doctors.) Instead, the letter stated: "The additional evidence which was submitted is not sufficient to warrant modification of the determination that the weight of medical evidence establishes that your employment related disability ceased by and not later than September 22, 1991, and compensation is terminated effective that date." Impressed by OWCP's apparent clairvoyance, I waited until September 21, but no miracle cure arrived.

That they terminated benefits did not surprise me. That they acknowledged receipt of the reports that actually pinpointed brain damage, yet concluded that the reports showed nothing new, did surprise me. Meanwhile, OWCP was liable for the charges for the data they were ignoring. I had spent $2,500 and round trip fare for the PET scan at the Brain Imaging Center in California. The neurologist-psychiatrist bills were substantial. He had come to Seattle to see me since I found that travel was a problem. None of those bills has been paid to this day, despite the fact that they were incurred during the time when medical expenses and compensation were due without question.

I had no choice but to go on disability retirement. It is noteworthy that the medical information I sent to the Office of Personnel Management to open my disability claim was the same information that OWCP had rejected. Based on the same data, disability retirement began. One government; two different perceptions of the same thing.

My monthly financial resources now changed dramatically. Under worker's comp, I had been due ⅔ salary without income tax plus medical expenses for the accepted condition. The change to disability retirement meant that I received less than $430 a month, subject to income tax.

It is ironic that OWCP seemed convinced I had concocted a plan to get income without work. Had that been my plan, I couldn't have made more mistakes.

The first "mistake," in this sense had occurred several years before my employment with the Corps, when I had left a job with the navy. To keep me going until I found new employment, I had withdrawn my retirement. At that time it was possible to withdraw that money and later pay it back — my intention — without having to pay interest. By the time of my poisoning, I had no way to pay the money back, and by then it could only be repaid with interest.

Next, I had taken a downgrade to work at the Corps, because I liked the agency and it was conveniently located. This caused my retirement to be set at GS-11, step 10, instead of its prior level of GS-12, step 6.

While I worked at the Corps, federal employees were offered the chance to change retirement programs. It was possible to remain on civil service retirement (CSR) or change to a program called FERS. I opted to remain on CSR.

The result of all these choices combined was that when chemical poisoning forced me to retire on disability, my retirement pay was so low that I could not live on it. FERS combined civil service retirement with social security. My choice prevented me from access to social security. Very poor planning, indeed.

The ending of 1991 was spent on odds and ends. In a letter dated September 9, 1991, my attorney responded to OWCP after having finally received the statement of accepted fact they had sent to the second referee doctor. He stated his objections to seven major points.

Recalling that the allergist to whom the consulting group had sent me had claimed to have run blood work on me, I sent a Freedom of Information request letter to the assistant director of OWCP in the Seattle district, asking for a copy of the report. The blood work was said to have been run by two labs, one in Seattle and one at Northwestern University. The Seattle report arrived, but the one from Northwestern University has never been produced. That violates the Freedom of Information Act.

I was trying to pursue a recommendation by the neurologist-psychiatrist who had sent me to California. He wanted me to have an evoked potentials brain map. The only way to deal with OWCP would be to provide medical data showing information they did not already have that supported the claim. I spent a lot of time hunting out a source for the test. I wanted someone who would do a pre-exposure test and then test me with a small amount of carpet glue to determine whether there was any effect from the exposure. I assumed that would provide better data, and I personally wanted to know. Finally, through conversations with other chemical sensitives, I located a practice that might have the equipment I needed to pursue the testing. I called the office and made an appointment.

The year 1991 would be a one that even with memory problems I'd gladly forget. I had seen some pretty awful things under the rocks I picked up, but this year revealed the ugliest ones yet. Quickly I was slipping into poverty. Yet I could not give up. The problem could be solved somehow. The order I gave myself was to try to solve it until I had done all I could do. That was a lot.

1992

My appointment with these new doctors was in January 1992. I explained what I had in mind and was delighted to discover that, in fact, they did have exactly what I needed. Both doctors decided to go ahead and test with challenge. I was amazed that it was so easy to persuade them. Little did I know that they had been waiting for someone like me to come along. They were eager to prove that MCS was psychogenic. They figured they could use their equipment to do just that. I had to laugh when one of the doctors suggested that the tests might not show anything. I assured him that the test would show plenty.

On another day I returned to the office to go over the test results. I was shocked when the doctor asked if he could retest me at his own expense. Reluctantly I agreed. Later I discovered the reason for his request. The findings were so abnormal that the doctor was convinced that the machine, which had just been serviced, was malfunctioning. When the second set of results were identical to the first set, the doctor was amazed. As I had predicted, he did find results.

That required him to make a tremendous readjustment. It was not easy. Doctors who change from one view to another are often condemned by the medical establishment. It takes a certain amount of guts to admit that one's previous view may have been mistaken. To do so when there is so much pressure to discount the reality of MCS requires great courage and integrity. These doctors had both.

The findings of the testing were significant. They demonstrated that even without exposure, my brain malfunctions. For example, it became clear that my ability to walk had been re-routed. The electrical impulses from my feet and hands reach the brain perfectly. Once there they are supposed to go to the motor cortex, a band that goes over the head roughly from ear to ear. My electrical impulses in the brain appear to avoid the motor cortex altogether, bouncing around my brain instead. In one case the right foot transmits to the hand part of the motor cortex on the wrong side of the brain. I would describe my ability to walk as a visual process. Following exposure the latency and amplitude of the electrical signals show delayed latency and in some cases (e.g., left leg) the signal flat-lines.

Other findings include:

- I hear what I see. The electrical signal goes from my eye to the visual cortex at the back of the head, as it should, but it also goes to the auditory cortex. The ringing in my ears is caused by my "hearing" the visual electrical signal.

- Following exposure to a tiny amount of carpet glue I see two images with my right eye and three with the left. Normal double vision is binocular. Mine is monocular. I have to adjust to seeing one thing. I cannot explain how I do it. At the time of this finding only one other person in medical literature is reported to have monocular double vision.

- If bright light hits my eyes, it floods my brain with voltage.

[174]

- Electrical signals make waves in the brain fluid. In my case, the explanation I got was that normal waves could be compared to the ripples a canoe would make on a lake; my waves, in comparison, would be made by an ocean liner.

- Short-term memory is affected by the hippocampal lesion, and in addition, the electrical signal gets to the storage part of the brain two to three times later than necessary to be stored.

The doctors studied these data for quite some time, then retested me before completing a final report. Both doctors make it clear that I am totally and permanently impaired. Work is out of the question. In the future I may be incapable of moving or communicating.

While this testing was going on, I chose to request another set of tests. The immunological data doctors first sought with MCS patients has run into so many obstacles that I wanted to know whether the challenge testing would show a concomitant change in my immunoglobulins.

A little background is helpful. My blood work showed TMA antibodies. Work done at the Environmental Protection Agency found that cases of poisoning associated with carpet were largely a function of the offgassing of styrene butadiene or 4-PC. It happens that these chemicals are very similar to TMA. TMA and styrene are almost chemically identical. If exposure to carpet glue, which is styrene butadiene, kicked off the immunoglobulin for TMA, that should tie back to the workplace exposure. It would show cross-reaction of TMA and styrene butadiene on the test. In addition to that, a literature search documented that rats exposed to styrene developed brain lesions identical to mine. I needed thorough documentation. At last I thought I could see progress. At least I had a far better understanding of my problems. The immune profiles did show that the styrene butadiene carpet glue set off TMA antibodies.

On September 14, 1992, my attorney filed a 200-page report with OWCP. We assumed we were filing in a timely matter. New medical evidence following termination should be filed within one year for reconsideration.

Some time during the summer or fall of 1992 I called one of the doctors in occupational medicine to whom I had been referred by my first pulmonologist. I wanted to tell him about the evoked potentials finding. Over the years he had expressed interest in my case, though he had told me that the pressure on doctors dealing with MCS was very great. He had always talked about wanting to know the truth with respect to MCS. I explained that he'd understand if he looked into the evoked potentials results. "Bonnye," he sighed, "you forced me into learning all I could about immunology. Now, you're telling me that I need to study neurology." I responded, "It comes with the territory."

On September 30, 1992, an employee at OWCP wrote a memorandum to the director in the case of Bonnye L. Matthews. Essentially it stated that the one-year period for requesting a reconsideration had begun on September 9, 1991— the date of the letter stating that termination was forthcoming. Termination had not begun until Sept. 22. Nevertheless, OWCP denied the application for reconsideration on the basis that the filing was not timely.

In the next day or two my attorney went to OWCP. He explained that the reconsideration pending was adequate to cover the date of the September 14 filing. He received assurance that the reconsideration would go forward.

In late October or early November, however, OWCP informed Mr. Sweeting that they refused to do the reconsideration. A conversation took place. The OWCP officials told Mr. Sweeting that they hoped I'd fire him. They thought I would blame him for failure to get the document "timely filed." If they had checked their records, they would have realized that Mr. Sweeting was working for nothing.

The OWCP officials also told Matt that they would never rule to put me back on the compensation rolls. They had a plan. They refused to rule on the reconsideration itself but chose instead to fail to act due to the "untimely" filing. They knew that decision would be overturned, but it would take years to do it. They'd force me into appeal after appeal. If the Employees Compensation Appeal Board (ECAB) ever overturned them, they'd put me back on the rolls, immediately send me out to one of their doctors, and remove me again. I could live in the appeals system. The OWCP knew better than my attorney or I that ECAB was backlogged not in months but rather in years.

Lack of appropriate oversight at OWCP is obvious. Were there oversight, the officials would not have been willing to say what they did to my attorney, even if they believed it.

On November 5, 1991, Mr. Sweeting filed an appeal at ECAB. In his transmittal letter he stated: "I would like to note that I have been told by [name of employee] at OWCP that the department 'cannot win at ECAB' regarding the clearly erroneous September 30, 1992, determination by OWCP."

At that point I (and my granddaughter, who was now living with me) was continuing to live on less than $430 a month. Without family support I'd have been on the streets. In large measure what OWCP officials did in 1991 was to transfer the government's financial responsibility for my workplace injury to my widowed mother. The effect of this action on my mother was to dissolve her financial resources while she carried a burden not hers. The effect on the U.S. citizen was that proof of the adverse health effect potential of styrene butadiene latex glue was hidden by OWCP in the ECAB office. It will remain hidden there, if all goes according to OWCP's plan. Of course, OWCP has made it clear that they have no responsibility to share information about adverse effects that they find in medical reports. That function belongs to another agency.

On December 9, 1992, OWCP Seattle district sent me a demand for repayment of severance pay. I had filed for a waiver, which OWCP refused to grant. I went to a consumer credit counseling service to try to figure out, with what income I had, how I would be able to pay back the severance pay at the $50 a month OWCP demanded. The counselor looked at my financial data and flatly stated that I didn't have enough to live on, let alone to pay out on anything else.

During 1992 there was activity on the state level that had profound and lasting effects.

On June 3, 1992, State Labor & Industries drew up a contract with the doctor who had performed my OWCP-ordered second referee exam. She was to "provide direct support to claims adjudication process, including such activities as reviewing industrial insurance claims; advising as to the quality of medical care; evaluating the relatedness of physical findings to diagnoses and treatment plans; and assisting in intervention when continuing treatment does not result in measurable improvement," and so on. For this she could be paid at a rate of $120/hour + $5/hour malpractice insurance and up to a maximum of $1,000 per day + mileage reimbursable at state rates for up to 140 miles a day. The condition was "up to ten (10) days per month, of which 6 days shall be in Olympia." The maximum amount payable was $135,000. That contract spanning 7/92 to 6/30/93, was amended for the 6/30/93 to 6/30/94 period to increase maximum amount payable to $330,000 with mileage from 140 to 160.

For this doctor to have been given a contract with provisions that she review claims seems to provide opportunity for conflict of interest. One could legitimately ask: Did she review her own medical reports?

Little pieces of information were coming together. Taken alone they meant nothing. When placed in a timeline, little by little, they began to pull together and explain some of the hindrances faced by chemically injured workers.

1993–1994

The year 1993 began on a dismal note. I filed bankruptcy on February 1. I was devastated. I'd lost my health, my career, my hope of returning to work, and my ability to cover my expenses. The one thing I had left was my integrity — until I had to file bankruptcy. Up until then I had struggled fiercely to pay my bills, a bit at a time. Now I was forced to discharge all my debt, and I felt I had lost my integrity. Included in the discharge was the severance pay.

I had to go to bankruptcy court downtown and face not only humiliation but also bad health effects. Despite the fact that OWCP received a notice of the meeting at bankruptcy court, they chose not to attend. The court official asked whether I expected OWCP to accept my case within the next two years. Well aware of the backlog of ECAB actions, I had to say that the answer was no.

On February 2, the doctor who had conducted my second referee exam wrote to Kenneth Martin, MD, Chairman, Industrial Insurance Advisory Committee, Washington State Medical Association. She complained about the tests doctors were using. She mentioned results of a study — the flawed study in which I had participated in 1990. (Data from that study should not have been released.) She focused her attention severely upon one doctor who was using the tests mentioned as appropriate in Boeing's IME protocol. She railed on and on. She accused doctors of practicing outside their specialties. This was rather like the pot calling the kettle black. She did just that in my medical report. She did that in the very letter in which she made those accusations against others. The tests were immunological and neurological. She has no certification in either field. Her objective was to get the Washington State Medical Board to reject the validity of the tests doctors were using. Apparently without further ado — and without asking how, as a specialist in occupational medicine, this doctor was qualified to evaluate immunological and neurological tests — the board took her advice and decided that the tests in the Boeing protocol were not reimbursable medical expenses. This increased the negative environment in the state toward chemical injury claims, since it was agreed that the state would not reimburse the tests most likely to show clear, significant results.

In May of 1993 I called ECAB to get a feel for the length of time it would take for them to act on my case. I was informed that they had not finished the 1992 appeals and that mine was number 339 in line for 1993. It would be a long time.

In July of 1993, the *Annals of Internal Medicine* published a paper entitled "Immunologic, Psychological and Neuropsychological Factors in Multiple Chemical Sensitivity." This was a report on the study in which I had participated in 1990.

When I saw the paper, I was outraged. If nothing else, the doctor in charge had taken all the patients he'd been given and decided to use them as a larger group of patients with diagnosed MCS. Nothing had been further from the truth.

The doctor and I had both been present when the patients' doctor talked about the division of the group. I called the doctor of the patient pool about the article. Was my memory giving me problems on this or did I accurately remember the division of the patients into three categories? He assured me my memory was not defective on that. He was writing to the *Annals*. The misinformation on the study group completely invalidated the results. No rocket science here. The *Annals* rejected the doctor's letter and mine. It didn't matter that both of us could attest to the lack of validity of the study results. Essentially, the *Annals* chose to stamp the imprimatur of good science upon bad science.

On August 4, 1993, the *Federal Register* printed the Environmental Protection Agency's draft report: "Principles of Neurotoxicity Risk Assessment." This document stated:

> A number of recently developed computerized imaging techniques for evaluating brain activity and cerebral/peripheral blood flow have added valuable information to the neurologic diagnostic process. These imaging methods include thermography, positron emission tomography, passive neuromagnetic imaging (magnetoencephalography), magnetic resonance spectroscopy, computerized tomography, doppler ultrasonography, and computerized EEG recording/analysis (brain electrical mapping).... Although the equipment for brain imaging is expensive and not portable, neuroimaging techniques promise to be valuable clinical and laboratory research tools in human neurotoxicology [page 41571].

This well-informed document contrasts sharply with policy documents of Washington State composed in the same year.

I say this based on action taken by the state in their draft of *Interim Agreement on Chemically Related Illnesses (CRI)* dated September 3, 1993. The *Interim Agreement* was designed for one purpose: it clarified the policy adopted in April that said the State would refuse payment for any of the following tests performed on chemically injured workers: "qEEG, PET scan, SPECT scan, evoked potentials, brain mapping, immunologic testing." The Washington State Medical Board thus ruled out tests which the *Federal Register* indicated were the most promising and which were outlined in the Boeing IME protocol. The *Interim Agreement* gave the impression that if a direct correlation between a chemical substance and a specific disease were not already part of medical knowledge, it could not exist. This is the same reasoning used during the time of Christopher Columbus: "No, you can't have a boat to do that! The earth is flat!"

After a year of continually checking on my case with ECAB, I finally got an answer in May 1994. ECAB overturned OWCP's decision that the medical package was not filed in a timely manner. They directed OWCP to decide whether they would do a reconsideration. I calculated that if OWCP refused, which they had already assured my attorney they would, I would have a wait of at least 12 years for any possible answer, because OWCP and ECAB could take decisions one tiny piece at a time. ECAB also directed me to repay severance pay. That seemed moot, since the debt had been discharged and OWCP had been sent a discharge notice.

By July 1994, my attorney had learned that not only had my file not been returned to OWCP, but it was split in half at ECAB and one half was missing. It took intervention from my Congressman, Mike Kreidler, to find the file at ECAB and send it to Seattle for action. The file arrived at OWCP Seattle district on September 9, 1994.

Matt had asked OWCP to process the reconsideration action expeditiously since the file had been missing at ECAB for such a long time. OWCP responded that they would make no extra effort. What that did was to place a 90-day timing on their decision as to whether to do a merit review (reconsideration of the neurological package).

On September 9, 1994, OWCP received a medical report informing them that the diagnosis of my medical condition had changed from MCSS to "…chemically induced porphyria with multiple deficits in the heme synthesis system, organic brain syndrome, and occupational asthma." The report went on: "This disease is separate from the hereditary porphyrias.... The disease has no cure.... Contact with substances which trigger attacks can lead to death.... If neurologic damage is done during an attack, the damage may become permanent."*

In a letter dated October 6, 1994, OWCP in Washington, D.C., demanded repayment of severance pay with interest. Action was threatened if I refused to comply. My attorney responded with a copy of the discharge order and Schedule F.

Meanwhile, the *Interim Agreement* of September 1993 was getting around. The fact that the Washington State government was willing to go along with such flat-world thinking gave much concern to others. Two doctors from the University of Pittsburgh were among the doctors who wrote to Mark Brown, Director, Washington State Department of Labor and Industries. The Pittsburgh doctors had the following comment on the *Interim Agreement*:

> In your draft of September 3, 1993 you state that one of your goals is "to assure that accurate diagnoses are made" (pg. 1). It seems that you are doing every thing in your power to not obtain accurate diagnoses. I hope that you and your committee members will weigh the evidence carefully before discounting years of research and clinical evidence in the field of medicine, psychiatry, psychology and occupational medicine.

This letter had no effect whatever.

On November 10, 1994, the end of OWCP's 90-day allowed period to decide whether they'd do the reconsideration merit review, Congressman Kreidler's office called OWCP to inquire about their decision. An OWCP employee agreed that the 90-day period had expired but explained that claims examiners are permitted a 10 percent error rate. The OWCP estimated the decision would take an additional 60 days.

Was OWCP playing politics? It was Congressional election time, and the race between Mike Kreidler and his opponent was too close to call. It seemed likely that OWCP did not want to make a decision until they knew whether Kreidler, who had an agenda for dealing with OWCP abuses, would be reelected.

On November 10, 1994, OWCP in Washington, D.C., wrote asking for proof from the attorney involved with bankruptcy that the Labor Department was properly served with the petition for bankruptcy. Attorneys have

---

*To review the complete report on the change of diagnosis, see the Appendix to this chapter, beginning on page 185.

no responsibility for proving that those papers were delivered. That was the job of the court.

Since my court file had been forwarded to archives in June 1994, we got the request out for bankruptcy court to provide the data. The court was able to act expeditiously. By November 19, 1994, I received the necessary proof.

Finally in a letter dated November 29, 1994, an official from the D.C. office of OWCP wrote to me:

> Please disregard my letter to you dated October 6, 1994. We will not be taking the actions indicated therein. Also, please be advised that we have written off the outstanding debt balance in your case on the basis that it has been discharged....

Had OWCP accepted my request for a waiver due to financial hardship, the government would not have wasted taxpayers' money pursuing its erroneous case against me. Furthermore, I could have avoided filing for bankruptcy, and my creditors would not have been forced to eat my debt, which I had been slowly repaying.

1995–PRESENT

Not until February 1, 1995, did OWCP respond to the ECAB decision of May 1994. The decision on reconsideration was, "The evidence submitted in support of the application is not sufficient to warrant modification of the prior decision." No explanation was given.

I was outraged. The neurological data from the brain map, which uses a P-300 brain wave known for not being affected by emotion (i.e., rules out psychogenic influence), was in the hands of OWCP along with the change to the specific porphyrinopathy diagnosis backed with clinical data. I was required to show that symptoms had not evaporated but rather had continued. I had submitted ample proof. Yet OWCP did exactly what they had assured my attorney that they would do: They returned me to the appeals process. It didn't matter that my claim was just. It didn't matter if my family and I lived in poverty. It didn't matter that the general public had no idea that glued-down carpet could be hazardous to one's health. Evidently nothing mattered to OWCP except the assurance that I would sit for years at ECAB, where the backlog grows and grows.

I knew what the disorder of porphyrin metabolism meant to me. The acute intermittent porphyria diagnosis was distasteful. AIP leads to death, and the end stages are not very pleasant to contemplate. The OWCP officials were playing games with my life. My health was deteriorating. I needed to see a dentist, but I couldn't afford it. I had asthma attacks, but I couldn't afford the machine that delivers the medicine in a way I can take it (nebulizer).

Ironically, that I am disabled has not been ignored by

- The U.S. Office of Personnel Management — they pay my disability retirement.
- The Internal Revenue Service — they provide the disabled credit.
- The State of Washington — they provide disabled parking.
- King County Superior Court — they excused me from jury duty.
- Local hospitals — they are extremely careful with me when I have to be there.

By the winter of 1996, my health had deteriorated to the point that it frightened me. Today I feel as if I am held together with tape and paperclips. Some of the things I could do to improve are beyond my ability. I do what I can. I wait.

POSTSCRIPT

As a problem solver I am frustrated when people in positions of authority leave me with the impression that the problems with OWCP are so large it would take an extraordinary effort just to get others to join to deal with the issue.

There is a far less complicated approach. First of all, it should be recalled that workers' compensation programs were developed to address a particular problem. Back at the turn of the century, courts were jammed with suits against employers. To free the litigation process, workers' comp took the no-fault approach, like some auto insurance policies today. Today, however, the no-fault perspective has been lost. A simple back-to-basics approach isn't unreasonable. Here's what I have in mind.

As soon as OWCP receives a claim from an injured employee, the claims examiner's first step should be to examine the doctor's certification to insure that he or she is in good standing with the state. If the medical report filed with the claim indicates the employee will be unable to work for two months, then compensation and medical expenses should begin immediately. That is in keeping with the idea of no-fault insurance. It also protects the employee against OWCP's current policy of permitting claims examiners (some of whom have no more than a high school education) to have greater authority over a claimant than the claimant's own treating physician.

If OWCP needs additional information, they could request it from the doctor in writing. The OWCP should send the doctor its list of criteria for continuing to accept long-term disability relating to the claimant's medical condition and point out specifically what appears to be lacking among the criteria. The OWCP should also request that the doctor send the claimant out for a second opinion. Right now, it is OWCP who refers the claimant out. That sets up the IME system, which is a corruption of proper medical doctor-patient interaction. If the second opinion agrees with the initiating doctor, OWCP should pay the claim without further question for one year (or the time the doctor thinks the employee may be able to return to work). If not, the OWCP should ask the initiating doctor to explain the differences in opinion. If the differences cannot be explained, OWCP should request the doctor refer out again. If the differences become reconciled in this manner, then the case should be set for one year follow-up (or the date when the doctor indicates the employee should be able to return to work). If differences appear irreconcilable, then test results should be weighed. If objective test results are compatible with initial findings, weight should be given to the opinion with the supporting data. If OWCP has any reason to believe that the doctor is not being straightforward, OWCP would be free to contact the state medical disciplinary board.

After the one-year period, OWCP should be able to determine from the doctor's reports whether the claimant is likely to recover enough to return to work. At that point OWCP should require from the treating doctor a well-reasoned report on whether the claimant is likely to be able to return to the workplace within the next year. In a no-fault system that should be all that is necessary to separate short-term disability from permanent disability. If at the end of the two-year period the doctor states that the employee cannot return to work of any kind at any point and provides well-reasoned support for this statement, then OWCP should recognize the permanent quality of the injury. Following that OWCP could, if necessary, require an annual report on the continuing impairment of the claimant.

This is simple claims handling. It is a far cry from the current arrangement where claims examiners second-guess doctors and put the lives of some claimants at risk.

Simple claims handling would trim the OWCP workforce. It would safeguard the health of injured workers. It would cut government expense because the opportunity for extended wrangling would be greatly reduced. There would be no need for the excessive amount of paper case file keeping. All of the activity could be automated. It would provide efficient and effective claims handling so that claimants would no longer have to wait excessive amounts of time to know OWCP's decision. ECAB's backlog would be reduced because the need for ECAB lies within the practices of OWCP officials. Medical practitioners would not be tempted to change from doctor to consultant for financial reward. Insurance companies would no longer have to carry the financial weight of payment for medical expense that is rightly the government's. Congressional representatives and senators would not have to use time to get answers for so many individual constituents. And the government would not be paying a fortune to try to block payment for what must be paid anyway. Cut out the game-playing, and expenses will decrease by themselves.

ADDENDIX TO CHAPTER 8: REVIEW OF DISABILITY AND CHANGE OF DIAGNOSIS FOR BONNYE MATTHEWS

In a letter dated August 29, 1989, the U.S. Department of Labor's Office of Workers' Compensation Programs (DOL/OWCP) accepted "as related factors of ... Federal employment: Temporary Aggravation of Mucosal Irritation and Multiple Chemical Sensitivity Syndrome" with respect to the claim of Bonnye Matthews. The acceptance of Multiple Chemical Sensitivity Syndrome was based on an exam by Drs. — and — .... The diagnosis was appropriate at the time.

A syndrome is a group of signs and symptoms related to one another which provides a basis for investigating an illness without knowing precise cause. In another letter (December 13, 1989) to OWCP from Drs. — and —, the major areas of symptoms experienced by my patient, Bonnye Matthews, were identified: respiratory, neuropsychological/cognitive, and gastrointestinal symptoms.

IV : Personal Experience with MCS

On September 9, 1991, OWCP removed approval of compensation and medical expenses for Bonnye Matthews because "the weight of medical evidence establishes that ... employment related disability ceased by and not later than September 22, 1991." Apparently the basis for this decision was a report from Dr. —. I have read that report. There are problems....

History — Problem Identification

There is always value in reexamining the entire history of a patient's case after time has passed. Based on information that Bonnye Matthews supplied you, there were standard office materials in her office. The building also included the Government Printing Office (GPO). Her work involved significant paperwork and copying both at the photocopier in the office and from duplication services at GPO. During her employment a glued down carpet and vinyl strips were installed in her work area (spring 1987). The carpet stayed damp for several days, noticed only because she removed her shoes and placed her feet on the wet carpet.

Chart 1 is a conservative overview of some of the chemicals that were part of the environment in which Bonnye Matthews worked. It should be noted that all of these chemicals are neurotoxic or porphyrinogenic or both. A significant number affect the respiratory system.

Chart 2 is a list of symptoms reported on Bonnye Matthews' "Employee Statement — History of Illness and Part of Body Affected." Chemicals capable of effecting such symptoms are included on the chart.

Chart 1

Some Chemicals in Office Environment:	Source:	Known Human Effects:
n-Hexane* (1)	felt-tipped pens printing inks	CNS depression CNS dysfunction Nervous system degeneration Respiratory problems
styrene**† (1,2)	photocopier toner & ink printing ink carpet + glue + backing	Central nervous system Respiratory system Eyes, skin

*neurotoxic; metabolite has greater neurotoxic potential
**neurotoxic
†currently known porphyrinogenic substances

[186]

Some Chemicals in Office Environment:	Source:	Known Human Effects:
	computer & monitor equipment	
butadiene** (1)	carpet backing carpet adhesive	Eyes Respiratory system Central nervous system
phthalates† (chemical group for trimellitic anhydride) (1, 2, 3)	adhesives carpet & backing floor preparation for glued carpet installation on concrete floors	Respiratory system Immune system
polychlorinated biphenyls**† (1, 2, 4, 5, 6)	adhesives inks carbonless paper	Respiratory system Skin Eyes Liver
toluene** (1)	printing ink cleaning products perfume rubber cement	Central nervous system Liver Skin
vinyl chloride**† (1, 4, 6)	plastics, photographic material, carpets, upholstery, paper	Liver, blood Central nervous system Lymphatic system

---

*neurotoxic; metabolite has greater neurotoxic potential
**neurotoxic
†currently known porphyrinogenic substances

NOTE: Parenthetical numbers by chemicals indicate citations for chemical sources and health effects. They are: (1) C. Wilson, *Chemical Exposure and Human Health,* McFarland 1993. (2) T. Colburn, "Developmental Effects of Endocrine-Disrupting Chemicals in Wildlife and Humans, *Environmental Health Perspectives,* Vol. 101 No. 4, October 1993 [These chemicals have been included because of their ability to mimic estrogen.] (3) M. Rivera et al., "Trimellitic Anhydride Toxicity: A Cause of Acute Multisystem Failure." *Archives of Internal Medicine* 1981; 141(8): 1071–1074 [In addition to TMA asthma this adds TMA as cause of respiratory failure, anemia, gastrointestinal bleeding.] (4) National Library of Medicine, U.S. Environmental Protection Agency: "Integrated Risk Information System — Porphyria," November 1994. (5) E. K. Silbergeld: "Role of Altered Heme Synthesis in Chemical Injury to the Nervous System," from *Mechanisms of Chemical-Induced Porphyrinopathies,* Annals of New York Academy of Sciences, 1987. (6) M. O. Doss: "Porphyrinurias and Occupational Disease," from *Mechanisms of Chemical-Induced Porphyrinopathies,"* Annals of the New York Academy of Sciences, 1987.

Chart 2

Symptoms	MCSS Symptoms	Porphyria Symptoms	Chemicals Capable of Effecting Symptoms
---------------From: Employee's Statement — History of Illness---------------			
systemic reaction to antibiotics		X	antibiotics
sinus congestion	X		n-hexane styrene butadiene
voice problems	X		trimellitic anhydride n-hexane styrene butadiene
difficulty concentrating	X	X	n-hexane styrene toluene
asthma	X		n-hexane phthalates
difficulty breathing	X		n-hexane butadiene polychlorinated biphenyls toluene trimellitic anhydride vinyl chloride
cough	X		butadiene trimellitic anhydride
abdominal pain	X	X	toluene
fatigue	X	X	n-hexane styrene butadiene vinyl chloride
weight loss	X	X	n-hexane
gastrointestinal	X	X	styrene butadiene polychlorinated biphenyls toluene phthalates vinyl chloride
near fainting	X	X	n-hexane

Symptoms	*MCSS Symptoms*	*Porphyria Symptoms*	*Chemicals Capable of Effecting Symptoms*
			styrene
			butadiene
			polychlorinated
			biphenyls
			vinyl chloride
sleeplessness	X	X	styrene
			toluene
rapid pulse	X	X	
rapid breathing	X		
ringing in ears	X		
tingling fingers	X	X	n-hexane
			toluene

-------------From: Employee's Statement — Part of Body Affected------------
(not repeating symptoms listed above)

wake up not breathing	X		
sore throat	X		butadiene
			phthalates
			styrene
			trimellitic anhydride
cramping intestines	X	X	
bleeding intestines	X		trimellitic anhydride
			vinyl chloride
nausea	X	X	butadiene
			n-hexane
			polychlorinated
			biphenyls
			styrene
			toluene
			trimellitic anhydride
			vinyl chloride
hands shake		X	toluene
inability to hold with			
hands (drop things)		X	
difficulty hearing	X		
ringing in ears	X		
upper abdominal pain	X	X	toluene

Chart 3

Medically Identified Symptoms	MCSS Symptoms	Porphyria Symptoms	Basis of Determination
Respiratory			
respiratory distress	X		observation; listening
chest pain	X*	X*	observation: EKG
occupational asthma	X		work removal/return trials; pulmonary function tests
not pre-existing			18 year known history [1, 5]
mild level prior to methacholine challenge			pulmonary function tests
moderate level airway reactivity/asthma following methacholine challenge	X		methacholine challenge pulmonary function test
tight chest	X		observation; listening
wheezing	X		observation; listening
respiratory problems	X		observation
pneumonia			x-ray
dry cough (2/14/91)			observation; listening
Central Nervous System			
nausea	X		observation
faintness	X	X	observation
loss of cognitive ability moderate range as of 5/22/90	X	X	neuropsychological assessments; evoked potentials testing
deterioration in intellectual capacity and functioning (2/14/91) "severe" level of impairment	X	X	neuropsychological assessments; evoked potentials testing
impaired short term memory	X	X	neuropsychological assessment; evoked potentials testing
impaired concentration	X	X	neuropsychological assessment;

---

*Assuming cardiac problems have been ruled out

Medically Identified Symptoms	MCSS Symptoms	Porphyria Symptoms	Basis of Determination
			evoked potentials testing
depleted energy	X	X	observation
intellectual dysfunction	X	X	neuropsychological assessment
organic brain syndrome	X	X	neuropsychological assessment; evoked potentials testing
neuropsychological problems	X	X	neuropsychological assessment
no psychiatric illness of pre-existing nature	X	X	observation
psychomotor retardation	X		observation
paucity of spontaneous gestures & facial expression			observation
no anxiety			observation
no psychotic thought			observation
no hallucinations or delusions; ideas of reference			observation
no systemic paranoid ideas			observation
workaholic			observation
no use of alcohol			observation
impaired attention	X	X	neuropsychological assessment
distractibility	X	X	neuropsychological assessment
difficulty learning	X	X	neuropsychological assessment
decreased ability to perform complex multiple tasks	X	X	neuropsychological assessment
unspecified psychiatric factors			opinion
clouded sensorium (2/14/91)	X	X	observation
difficulty expressing self (2/14/91)	X	X	observation evoked potentials testing

Chart 3 (cont.)

Medically Identified Symptoms	MCSS Symptoms	Porphyria Symptoms	Basis of Determination
aphasia	X		evoked potentials testing; observation
disorientation	X	X	observation
agitation	X	X	observation
toxic encephalopathy	X	X	PET scan evoked potentials testing
brain damage in left hippocampus	X	X	PET scan; evoked potentials testing
frontal lobe assymetry	X	X	evoked potentials testing
balance defects	X	X	evoked potentials testing
muscular weakness	X	X	evoked potentials testing
vascular disease of brain	X		SPECT scan

Gastrointestinal

nausea	X	X	observation
gastrointestinal problems	X	X	observation, abdominal ultrasound, colonoscopy

Eyes

edematous eyelids	X		observation
vision problems	X	X	observation, evoked potentials test
monocular double triple vision			evoked potentials testing

Ears, Nose, Throat

nasal congestion	X		observation
hoarseness	X		observation
laryngeal edema	X		observation
dry cough (2/14/91)	X		observation

Medically Identified Symptoms	MCSS Symptoms	Porphyria Symptoms	Basis of Determination
deviated septum			observation, CAT scan
no deviated septum			observation
Circulatory			
chest pain	X*	X*	observation; EKG
tachycardia	X		pulse
vascular disease of brain	X		SPECT scan
low blood pressure	X		test
high blood pressure	X		test
Metabolic			
weight loss	X	X	observation
drug hypersensitivity	X	X	observation after administration
depleted energy	X	X	observation
Immune System			
TMA antibodies	X		immune test
autoantibodies	X		immune test
atopy	X		skin test
drug hypersensitivity	X	X	observation following administration
sensitivity	X	X	skin test

*Assuming cardiac problems have been ruled out

NOTE 1: Medical principle would value basis for determination in the following manner: evoked potentials testing (highest value: it uses the P-300 brain wave, a test that cannot be affected by emotion); clinical testing especially when performed with challenge (e.g., pulmonary function, PET scan, SPECT scan, porphyrins and their associated enzymes, neuropsychological assessment); observation; opinion (lowest value)

Chart 3 is a medical view of the symptoms listed on Chart 2. It is a composite of all the symptoms identified by doctors who examined Bonnye Matthews. Beside the symptom is the method by which the determination was made. This is critically important because there is mention in these medical reports in some cases that multiple chemical sensitivity syndrome is not a proven diagnosis. Consequently, proof whenever possible should accompany a diagnosis.

Chart 4 is the symptoms noticed by Bonnye Matthews' supervisor.

Although he was not medically trained, he was able to see two of the three major symptom areas (respiratory problems and cognitive problems [i.e., neuropsychological abnormalities]).

Chart 4
Symptoms Observed by Supervisor at Work

Difficulty breathing
Face flushed
Not thinking clearly

Until the end of 1994 classification of the problems at this point should have been:

1. occupational asthma
2. chemical sensitivity (or multiple chemical sensitivity syndrome)
3. toxic encephalopathy (or organic brain syndrome secondary to chemical exposure)

Bonnye Matthews has a real, not psychogenic problem. In addition to facing life with total, permanent disability, she has had to deal with a tremendous amount of stress. I have included an appendix in which she has chronicled that stress over several years. The stress and its effect on a disabled person should be considered.

Present—Diagnosis

In the summer of 1993 I ordered a CT scan for Bonnye Matthews due to serious sinus trouble. The increased problem traced back to the previous November, though there had been sinus congestion symptoms occurring back in the work environment. Bonnye Matthews does not tolerate antibiotics. The two newer ones, ceftin and biaxin, are very expensive. I would prescribe them for the sinus problem, and occasionally she would not fill them due to lack of money. With the CT scan information, however, I referred her to South Seattle Otolaryngology where she saw Dr. —. The condition was serious enough that surgery was required.

During the pre-surgery workup at Highline Hospital, when Bonnye Matthews was escorted to the lab for blood testing, she had a significant asthma attack in the area of the old lobby. In addition to asthma, she had difficulty walking. The hospital was having a carpet installed in the entryway to the old lobby. Escaping vapors triggered the attack before she could see what was occurring.

She was taken to the lab in a wheelchair. Following the blood testing she was taken for a standard EKG. The results of the EKG were abnormal. She had to be cleared by a cardiologist before surgery could take place. This is just one more piece of evidence in this case of what precipitates these asthma attacks.

It takes a long time to diagnose properly a case as complicated as this one. For those of us studying this syndrome seriously, the answer lay within our grasp, but it was clouded by one word: "hereditary." The obvious precipitating agent was environmental chemicals commonly in low doses. Who would think to look at a primarily hereditary disease noted for its rare incidence when faced with hundreds of patients whose symptoms are obviously tied to chemical exposure?

The answer lies in chemically induced porphyria (disorders of porphyrin metabolism). On Charts 1 to 3, there are references to porphyrinogenic substances and symptoms. The parallels between the sets are remarkable. In Chart 2, for example, Bonnye Matthews' symptoms listed in the material she put together for her January 1989 OWCP claim show striking parallels between those thought to be MCSS and those known to be porphyria. Even more striking are the data if the occupational asthma elements are removed. Chemicals that are known to produce her symptoms (neurotoxic and porphyrinogenic) are listed to the side. This is not coincidental. It results from observation, testing, and staying with it until proper answers are found. This cannot be done in an hour's IME.

Before going too far into the diagnosis of porphyria, it is important to pull together one final element. OWCP removed Bonnye Matthews from compensation indicating that by September 22, 1991, her disability would cease. It can only be assumed that the basis of such an action was that Dr. — was not able to see the symptoms and OWCP ignored the report from Dr. —. I have listed the initial presenting symptoms and the present symptoms in Chart 5. They are the same. What differs is that some are chronic and some are acute intermittent. Chronic symptoms are ones that should be observable constantly and the others vary in ability to observe.

As noted on the chart, acute intermittent symptoms are the ones which are the most likely to be life threatening. The disability did not cease.

Chart 5
Symptoms* from Initial Presentation to Present

	Initial Presentation	Present	Comments
Systemic reactions to antibiotics	X	X	acute intermittent
Sinus congestion	X	X	chronic
Voice problems	X	X	acute intermittent
Difficulty concentrating	X	X	chronic
Asthma	X	X	acute intermittent
Difficulty breathing	X	X	acute intermittent
Cough	X	X	acute intermittent
Abdominal pain	X	X	acute intermittent
Fatigue	X	X	chronic
Weight loss	X	X	acute intermittent
Gastrointestinal problems	X	X	acute intermittent
Near fainting	X	X	acute intermittent
Sleeplessness	X	X	acute intermittent
Rapid pulse	X	X	chronic
Rapid breathing	X	X	acute intermittent
Ringing in ears	X	X	chronic
Tingling fingers	X	X	acute intermittent
Wake up not breathing	X	X	acute intermittent
Sore throat	X	X	acute intermittent
Cramping intestines	X	X	acute intermittent
Bleeding intestines	X	X	acute intermittent
Nausea	X	X	acute intermittent
Hands shake	X	X	acute intermittent
Hands drop things	X	X	chronic
Difficulty hearing	X	X	chronic
Upper abdominal pain	X	X	acute intermittent

*Symptoms listed in Chart 2

NOTE: Acute intermittent classifications above are associated with low level toxic chemical exposures. The danger in acute intermittent reactions is that they are the most likely to generate life-threatening situations.

Considering the potential for porphyria, I have used the laboratory at Mayo's for extensive testing. Mayo's findings are: "Normal values for this patient's urinary and fecal porphyrins and porphyrins in erythrocytes and the diminished activity of the erythrocyte porphobilinogen deaminase suggest this case to be one of acute intermittent porphyria." The blood work shows that enzyme levels vary, characteristic of chemically induced (non-hereditary) porphyria. She also shows traits for porphyria cutanea tarda and coproporphyria. These atypical readings are foreign to some labs where only hereditary porphyrias are evaluated and only one enzyme is tested. Nationally, Mayo's Lab receives the difficult porphyria cases at a rate of approximately 800 a month. Because the enzyme levels and porphyrins from this patient vary directly in relation to toxic chemical exposure instead of remaining constant, the diagnosis preferred by Mayo's is chemically induced porphyria with multiple deficits in the heme synthesis system. It is separate from the hereditary forms of porphyria.

Generally, genetic defects create a single enzyme deficiency that remains at a stable level. Generally, toxic induced defects create multiple enzyme deficiences that vary in level dependent upon toxic exposure. Together, chemically induced porphyrinuria and multiple enzyme deficiency have led to clinical disease in this case. Tests combined with symptoms provide the proof.

Bonnye Matthews' tests and symptoms show clinical disease. Four high urinary porphyrins have been identified along with four low enzymes the latter of which vary dependent on toxic exposure (e.g., carpets, certain perfumes, printer toners, vehicle exhaust concentrations, tight buildings, downtown air, drugs, detergents, solvents, numerous metals, and so on).

Symptoms are consistent with acute intermittent porphyria rather than other hepatic porphyria presentations due to the neurologic component (organic brain syndrome, paresthesias, etc.). Skin, for example, is not significantly affected although the trait for porphyria cutanea tarda is present and the symptom of solar skin eczema is present. Photosensitivity which one might expect with coproporphyria is not present even during acute phases. She has significant problems with drugs which are known to be porphyrinogenic one instance in which the effect was life threatening. Specific drug problems include antibiotics, an antidepressant, an estrogen trial, aerosol inhalants, oral steroids, and others.

When Bonnye Matthews went to work at the U.S. Army Corps of Engineers, she was a normal, healthy individual, a productive worker. Following installation of a glued down carpet in the workplace, she experienced for the first time a life threatening systemic reaction to an antibiotic. She developed nasal congestion and chronic sinusitis. A few months after the carpet installation she papered the walls with post it boards so she "could put her brains on the wall." She had voice problems. Symptoms were developing obvious more readily by hindsight. Not until an explosive reaction occurred did she realize there was a significant problem.

Standard work removal/return trials removed any doubt as to the source of the problem. The significant amount of porphyrinogenic substances in that environment add further confirmation of the office as the source. Many people live full lives without ever developing clinical porphyrias when susceptibility is anticipated by family history. There certainly was no evidence of family susceptibility in this history. In this case it is highly probable that without work exposure to porphyrinogenic/neurotoxic substances at Federal Center South Bonnye Matthews might never have shown any signs of porphyria and could have continued a productive work history.

Without question Bonnye Matthews was poisoned by the carpet installation and the other porphyrinogenic substances in the workplace. That poisoning resulted in occupational asthma and chemically induced porphyria (ICD Code 277.1) with organic brain syndrome (ICD Code 294.9). Once clinical disease occurs, there is no cure. It is permanent. This disease will probably continue to progress because it is caused by contact with common chemicals. Nervous system damage at this point will generate symptoms of the acute attack. Outcomes of an attack can vary from death to recovery. Nervous system damage from which the patient recovers will include further deficits from the damage from which recovery is not likely. During attacks, vital capacity should be measured frequently when motor neuropathy is present. There is danger of death from rapidly progressing ventilatory insufficiency. The only treatment for this metabolic disorder is avoidance of porphyrinogenic and neurotoxic substances.

It should be noted that there have been suggestions that Bonnye Matthews receive counseling and pharmacologic treatment for possible masked anxiety/depression. Although it is clear that anxiety/depression is not the problem, there is good reason to avoid such suggestions in the future. Drugs commonly used in dealing with depression, anxiety, and psychosis are largely porphyrinogenic. It is reasonable to suspect that such treatment could be life threatening if not deadly.

Due to the ubiquity of porphyrinogenic and neurotoxic substances, this condition is totally disabling. For her to place herself in any situation where porphyrinogenic substances exist can at this point prove lethal. She is totally and permanently disabled.

ABOUT THE
CONTRIBUTORS

Eileen R. McCarty is a clinical psychologist in the Seattle area. Her work as early as the 1980s led physicians to consider the possibility of organic brain syndrome as the outcome of low-level toxic exposure. Testing by neuropsychologists has consistently supported her conclusions.

Donald L. Dudley, M.D., is a retired professor of psychiatry and behavioral sciences and former clinical professor of neurological surgery at the University of Washington. His findings on olfaction and chemical injury have been presented to the Society for Neurosciences and the Center for Disease Control Seminar on the Chemical Impact Project.

Gunnar Heuser, M.D., Ph.D., F.A.C.P., is a physician in Agoura Hills, California, with a practice in neurotoxicology and immunotoxicology. He is a fellow of the American College of Physicans and the American EEG Society, a diplomate (McGill University) in internal medicine, and a diplomate of the American College of Forensic Examiners.

Randolph I. Gordon, a 1978 graduate of the Harvard University School of Law, is an attorney in Bellevue, Washington, with a practice specializing in toxic tort litigation. In 1995 he successfully argued for injured workers in *Birklid v. Boeing*, a case before the Washington State Supreme Court. The resulting decision, for the first time in 73 years, permitted injured workers to go to a jury on the question of deliberate intent to cause injury in the workplace.

INDEX

Index

Index